Praise for Sacred Pregnancy

"Few women are so committed to advocating for a woman's right to birth her baby in a sacred and empowering way as Anni Daulter is. She has a tremendous gift to offer us all in her passion to protect the family dynamic as she shares the mysteries of the birth journey with us."

　—*Aleksandra Evanguelidi,* LM, CPM, owner of The Sanctuary Birth & Family Wellness Center

"*Sacred Pregnancy* is a wonderful book and is absolutely beautiful and touching. It really speaks to vital pregnancy issues—I would recommend this as a gift for all pregnant moms."

　—*Shiva Rose,* actress

"*Sacred Pregnancy* is an amazing book and it's so gorgeous! I wish this were available to me during any of my three pregnancies, as I think this will help women get more in touch with themselves throughout this beautiful process. I would happily recommend *Sacred Pregnancy* to all expecting moms."

　—*Shanna Moakler,* actress, TV personality, and mother of Alabama, Atiana, and Landon

"I am in LOVE with *Sacred Pregnancy*. I devoured it like it was food! I think every woman should carry it throughout her pregnancy. When a woman discovers she is pregnant, it can be a happy but overwhelming time. This book addresses all of the fears, concerns, myths, joys, rites, and relationships t⟨...⟩ come with pregnancy. Each thoughtful chapter has a dedicated ⟨...⟩ that particular topic, at once creating not jus⟨...⟩ n amazing keepsake of such a mag⟨...⟩

Filled with poignan⟨...⟩ inspiration, it takes you on a spiritual journe⟨...⟩ of pregnancy, encouraging you to revel in the awe of the unive⟨...⟩, your blossoming body, babies, and the awesome power of birth."

　—*Melanie Monroe,* Ecobaby Planning and Concierge

OTHER BOOKS BY ANNI DAULTER

Organically Raised: Conscious Cooking for Babies and Toddlers

Ice Pop Joy

The Organic Family Cookbook

Naturally Fun Parties for Kids

2-in-1: Feeding Your Baby, Feeding Your Family

Sacred Pregnancy

Sacred

FOREWORD BY *Ina May Gaskin*

FOREWORD BY *Anna Getty*

PHOTOGRAPHY BY *Elena Rego and Alexandra DeFurio*

Pregnancy

A Loving Guide and
Journal for Expectant Moms

ANNI DAULTER, MSW

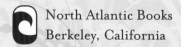

North Atlantic Books
Berkeley, California

Published by
North Atlantic Books
P.O. Box 12327
Berkeley, California 94712

Cover photo by Elena Rego and Alexandra DeFurio
Cover and book illustrations by Sam & Abigail Alfano
Cover and book design by Claudia Smelser
Printed in the United States of America

Sacred Pregnancy: A Loving Guide and Journal for Expectant Moms is sponsored by the Society for the Study of Native Arts and Sciences, a nonprofit educational corporation whose goals are to develop an educational and cross-cultural perspective linking various scientific, social, and artistic fields; to nurture a holistic view of arts, sciences, humanities, and healing; and to publish and distribute literature on the relationship of mind, body, and nature.

North Atlantic Books' publications are available through most bookstores. For further information, visit our website at www.northatlanticbooks.com or call 800-733-3000.

MEDICAL DISCLAIMER: The following information is intended for general information purposes only. Individuals should always see their health care provider before administering any suggestions made in this book. Any application of the material set forth in the following pages is at the reader's discretion and is his or her sole responsibility.

The Library of Congress Cataloging-in-Publication Data is available from the publisher upon request.

2 3 4 5 6 7 8 9 UNITED 16 15 14 13 12

Sacred Pregnancy is dedicated to my husband, Tim, who has supported me through every birth and to my children Zoe, Lotus, Bodhi, and River, whom I love more than words can ever express. This book is also dedicated to all women who cross over that threshold from maiden to mother with confidence, awareness, and the fierce energy it takes to guide their children through life.

℅ ANNI DAULTER

For the conscious sacred mamas out there who hold the heart space for life to come forth, both physically and spiritually.

℅ ELENA REGO

For my Mooshkie and Sugar Pie. You both made me the luckiest Mama around! I love you, my sweet angel girls!

℅ ALEXANDRA DEFURIO

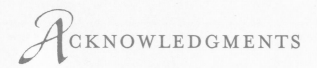ACKNOWLEDGMENTS

First, I want to say to my mother, thank you so much for bringing me into the world at such a young, ripe age of seventeen, full of fear in unknown territory. You birthed me and carried me on your back through the forest and led me to my path of lifelong discovery. You are my role model and I love you. Thank you, Mama.

To my husband, Tim, who has made me a mother many times over and who always supports everything I do. Thank you for believing in this vision and making copies in the middle of the night to mail out to publishers in hopes someone else would see our vision too. You are a brave dad and my champion and have stood by me at every home birth and held my hand. I love you.

To my kiddos. Zoe, Lotus, Bodhi, and River Love ... I adore you and every day I get to spend with each of you is such a treasure. Thank you for the many reminders you give me to stay in my higher self so that I can help guide you down your right path in life. Lotus, you are my angel. Zoe, you are my hope. Bodhi, you are my laughter, and River, you are my joy.

To Sally, my agent and friend. I am so blessed to have found you and want to thank you for seeing what this project could be from the moment you first saw it. You did not give up and you found the perfect home for it! I am so grateful.

To everyone, especially Elizabeth and Claudia, at North Atlantic Books and Random House for believing in this project and pushing to get it made!

To Elena and Alexandra, say what? We finally pulled this off! I can hardly believe it gals, but after all the meetings, chats, and talks about the vision, this project has finally manifested itself. This has been a labor of love and your gorgeous photography is stunning and moving. I am so grateful that both of you threw yourself into this book. I love you both so dearly!

To Cristy, thank you so much for coming through at the last minute and sharing your photos with us. You are amazing and the work you do brings tears to my eyes.

To Dr. Biter, for all you do to protect birth for women and for being the change you want to see in the world.

To my midwives over the years (Catherine, Aleks, and Jake) and all midwives, who help nurture and support women through their pregnancies and births. You amaze me and you make births magical and help empower women, and for that I honor you.

To my dear friends, sisters, and supporters: Tnah, Amy, Kelly, Ann, Tree, Jen, Rachel, Nikki, Luann, Anna Getty, and Alisa, for all your work with Pregnancy Awareness Month. To Christy Funk, for all you do to support women and babies. To my circle sisters: Ellen, Tara, Cari Ellen, Tara B., Jackie, Jennifer, and Peggy. To all the models who came out and agreed to be a part of this vision, and to Ina May Gaskin for being awesome and supporting this book and for her work in the world.

To my in-laws, Bonnie and Dan, for all the love and support and for watching the kids so I could get the book done!

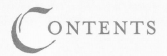

CONTENTS

FOREWORD *by Ina May Gaskin*   x

FOREWORD *by Anna Getty*   xii

INTRODUCTION   *Welcome to Sacred Pregnancy*   xiv

Week 1   Journal 1

Week 2   Sacred Space 9

Week 3   Due Date 17

Week 4   Meditation 25

Week 5   Cravings 33

Week 6   Womb 41

Week 7   Expectations 49

Week 8   Body Image 57

Week 9   Romance 65

Week 10   Birth Art Expression 73

Week 11   Exercise 81

Week 12   Mindful Eating 89

Week 13   Radiant Glow 97

Week 14   Bonding 105

Week 15   Partner Energy 113

Week 16   Sexy Mama 121

Week 17   Joyfulness 127

Week 18   Nurturing Yourself 133

Week 19   Fear 139

Week 20   Forgiveness 147

Week 21   Movement Within 155

Week 22   Trust 161

Week 23   Baby Girl 169
Week 24   Baby Boy 177
Week 25   Love 185
Week 26   Earth Energy 193
Week 27   Air Energy 199
Week 28   Fire Energy 205
Week 29   Water Energy 213
Week 30   Nesting 221
Week 31   Adornment 233
Week 32   Blessingway 241
Week 33   Naming Ceremony 249
Week 34   Visualization: Your Perfect Birth 257
Week 35   Empowerment 265
Week 36   Sisterhood Connection 273
Week 37   Surrender 281
Week 38   Surges 289
Week 39   Birth 297
Week 40   Rite of Passage 307

BIRTH STORIES   *314*

RESOURCES   *321*

WHY I OPENED A BIRTHING CENTER, *by Dr. Robert Biter, MD*   *325*

STAGES OF LABOR   *327*

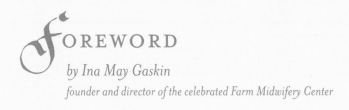

Traditional societies have typically regarded pregnancy as a sacred period in a woman's life—a time when the pregnant woman must be treated with special care and reverence by the other members of her society. As the carrier of new life, she embodies the miracle of creation in her very being, linking the generations with her every breath. Pregnancy confers upon her a special status in these societies that simultaneously determines how everyone treats her and also lays out special tasks and responsibilities that she has to attend to in a conscientious way throughout her pregnancy. Such preparation and conscientiousness greatly increase the chances that both she and her baby will safely come through the passage of labor and birth. Equally important, the mother's best interests and those of her baby are not seen as antithetical to each other.

Indigenous societies value women's ability to give birth and work to ease women's passage into new motherhood. In such societies, people make special efforts not to harass or frighten pregnant women about the process of labor and birth. Far from it. Such human groups have no ulterior motive that would induce them to attempt to scare women when the subject of birth is raised (such as the profit motive of a corporate health-care industry, or the need to create a more exciting and dramatic birth story to attract the attention of an audience).

Our mainstream U.S. culture, on the other hand, has for more than a century regarded birth primarily as an event that separates mother and baby. The separation is the most important part, and it is often assumed that anything good that happens with the mother in this process can't possibly good for the baby. Within this framework, culture negates and debases the idea that birth should be regarded as a sacred event, emphasizing instead its risks and dangers even when birth goes perfectly well. In discussions in which the sacred nature of pregnancy and birth is brought up, the answer often presumes that anything that would revalue the sanctity of birth would automatically put babies in danger. Nothing could actually be farther from the truth.

Can a sacred valuation of pregnancy and birth exist in a technological society? Anni Daulter is betting that it can, and I'm with her. Her book is beautifully designed to help you learn how to trust your beautiful, creative body at the same time that you prepare yourself in an optimum way for labor and birth. She invites you to take pride in your body's ability, and to believe in its ability to do whatever it needs to do in birth—even when that is still somewhat mysterious to you. *Sacred Pregnancy* invites us to create such a space in our modern lives, to honor what is beautiful and sacred about a woman's power to create life.

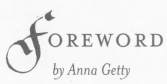

FOREWORD

by Anna Getty

founder of Pregnancy Awareness Month and happy home–birther of two

In twenty-first century America, pregnancy and birth have intersected at a point between disconnection and trendiness. Let me explain. Once upon a time women went into pregnancy supported by their community. It may not have been a glamorous time, but back then women stood beside pregnant and birthing mothers. Babies came onto the planet much of the time with midwives, grandmothers, aunts, and sisters guiding them out of the womb. This was a rite of passage. It was real and raw and natural.

Later pregnancy and birth were taken out of the hands of women and somehow redesigned to fit into "a man's world" by becoming an anaesthetized, clinical business. This is still the trend. For the most part this format also encompasses viewing the baby as an accessory. Women and men want the baby shower, the gear, the pretty little nursery and cute clothing as well the pain-free, clean, and convenient birth, all the while forgetting that when a women gets pregnant, she has the opportunity not only to birth a baby but rebirth herself as well.

These parents-to-be march into parenthood relatively unprepared and missing a point: that pregnancy and birth are actually divine and sacred moments in a woman's life. In *Sacred Pregnancy,* Anni Daulter reminds us that we have a tremendous opportunity to delve into a profound place within ourselves during pregnancy and birth. We have to take back the power of birthing and surrender to our natural, creative essence. Birth is creation, and this book is the foundation of creating the community we deserve and desire during this vulnerable and delicious time.

Delve into your process week by week, unlocking the beauty inside you. Feel the fear, the excitement, the uncertainty, the tenderness, and the courage that will arise in you. Allow yourself to be guided, to experience your conscious and sacred birth. It is your birthright.

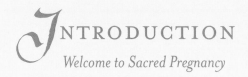

INTRODUCTION
Welcome to Sacred Pregnancy

Being pregnant and giving birth are like crossing a narrow bridge. People can accompany you to the bridge. They can greet you on the other side. But you must walk the bridge alone.

AFRICAN PROVERB

If you have picked up this book, and found yourself called to read it, know that there is a reason and trust that. You don't have to know right away why the book spoke to you, just take your time with it and the reason will likely unfold for you at some point throughout this process. Creating a new life brings about many changes, both physical and emotional. And this book is here as an inspirational resource, a good friend, and a practical guide to help you through your personal process of becoming a mother. In today's Western cultures, the typical pregnancy resources focus heavily on the growth of the baby, often to the exclusion of the woman herself. *Sacred Pregnancy* was written to help you through this journey by inviting you to explore yourself as you prepare for the birth of your baby. It is meant to honor your personal journey as you grow emotionally through the many transitions of your pregnancy, and to offer you vital information on how your baby is physically developing week to week and how that process can be impacting your body and spirit. My wish is that you feel empowered to create the birth experience that you desire and walk into it with confidence, strength, and a deeper understanding of this woman's work of birthing your baby.

Although it's fun and exciting to prepare for your new baby by buying infant-related items, decorating a nursery, and taking birthing classes, it is equally important to slow down and consider what is going on emotionally for you. Your body is changing, your emotions are spiraling, and your relationship with your partner is shifting. Introspection is critical as you prepare to step across the threshold to motherhood. There was a time when women gathered with their sisters and experienced pregnancy in a sacred way, when stories were passed down from elder women to young mothers. They were taught how to embrace pregnancy with reverence and to honor the first breaths of life as their babies entered the world. Today, women have to search to find this type of support and many women end up facing the roller coaster of pregnancy feeling very alone. Based on this book, Sacred Pregnancy class series are being offered. There are Redefining Pregnancy circle series and Redefining Birthing circle series popping up around the country. Please visit the Sacred Pregnancy website (www.sacredpregnancy.com) to join a group in your area or to learn more about how to become a certified Sacred Pregnancy instructor and lead your own circle series. No pregnant woman should have to feel alone during such a life-altering experience. As this book becomes a trusted friend, know that there are resources and communities out there that will support you as you walk this amazing pathway. When you feel empowered to make critical choices throughout your pregnancy and you make those decisions in full awareness, you will start motherhood with confidence and glory and know that your child is damn lucky to have a mother like you!

This book is deeply personal to me and it took my photographers, Elena and Alexandra, and me three years to prepare. We are dedicated to it because we believe this book has a real purpose in the hands of pregnant women and birthing communities, and we are very proud of what we have created. We hope that this book truly becomes a trusted friend throughout this pregnancy and are grateful you came along for the ride.

In gratitude, Anni

How to Use This Book

For forty weeks, this book will travel with you, as you experience mood swings, intense feelings, and body changes. Each week there will be important pregnancy tips and information on your baby, your body, and your spirit that correspond to a particular topic for deeper exploration. Each topic is accompanied by a gorgeous photo, reflections, ideas, and journal pages designed to help you relate to the specific topic and its meaning. The journal section following each topic description will allow you to take time to record your thoughts and feelings, including any reactions to the images, reflections, and meditations. This book can also serve as a memory keepsake for sharing stories and insights from your pregnancy with your child as she grows up.

Create a Pregnancy and Birthing Support Team and Build Your Sisterhood Circle!

It is important to create a support system for yourself in the beginning of your pregnancy so you have folks to call on when you are in need. This includes the VERY important decision of choosing a practitioner. You may already have an OB-GYN whom you see and who you always thought would always assist in your births. You may, however, want to try a midwife. This is a very personal decision for you and your partner and should not be stepped into lightly. Do your research and think about what kind of birth experience *you* want. When you get pregnant, especially if you have questions about alternative birthing options, I recommend you watch *The Business of Being Born* video, produced by Ricki Lake and Abby Epstein. Have you always been curious about folks who have home births or birthing-center births? Do you secretly wish you could do it if you had more support? These are good questions to ask yourself as you plan this experience. You may also opt for having both a midwife and an OB-GYN. You can always see a midwife along with your OB-GYN appointments. I know it's "double-dipping," but it may make you feel more comfortable. There are there are amazing midwives doctors out there who do support women in their power to birth, like Dr. Robert Biter, who by the way is also becoming a midwife just so he can see that side of the story! Look around and you will find the right person for you.

My first child, born fourteen years ago now, was born at a birthing center. Right after I found out I was pregnant, I did what most women in the U.S. do, I made an appointment with my OB-GYN. I will never forget how excited I was to be there and to have an opportunity to ask her my million questions. I remember sitting in the cold, little office going over all the questions I had in my head. The doctor came in and quickly said, "you are due November 8 and you need to make a monthly appointment to see me. You can do that when you leave." She then began to walk out of the room, while looking at her watch, and with one foot out the door, turned over her shoulder and asked, "Do you have any questions?" I thought, "Yeah, I do, but clearly they are not going to be answered here by you." I left that day hoping and praying there was another option for my prenatal care and vowed never to step foot in that office again.

The next week I had an appointment with a midwife, who spent two hours—yep, two whole hours—answering ALL of my questions. Of course this was all done in her lovely office sitting on a comfy couch, while sharing tea and starring in awe at all of the beautiful images that hung on the walls of powerful women birthing their babies. Those two hours changed my life path and ultimately led me here, and to writing this book. I knew if those women on her walls could do it, then so could I. I knew that I was part of a tribe, a lineage of women who were empowered enough to create their own birthing experiences despite the fear mongering of the medical community. After successfully birthing my nine-pound son Zoe in the birthing-center bathtub, I realized I could have just as easily done that at home and vowed that next time I would not bother wasting time traveling to someone else's tub. I would just stay in the warmth of my own nest to birth my babies. Seven years later, my daughter Lotus was born at home with another midwife. Two years after that, my third child Bodhi was born at home and two years later, my fourth child River was born at home "in the caul" (with his water sack still intact). Having had four babies with loving midwives and doulas present for support, I know that I would not want to bring my children into the world any other way. I believe this is how women are meant to birth, with other women, in loving, supportive environments, with freedom and no stress, and, most importantly, with people around her who share the belief that she can do it. In the moment of birthing a baby, she is the most powerful woman in the world. I experienced that four times over, and I am grateful, as I found what was best for me. What is the most important thing for *you* to do, as you begin down this path of deciding who you want to help support you in this process, is to be educated and empowered so you are fully aware of the birthing options before you and your partner decide which birthing route to travel. Don't be afraid of birth; instead be empowered and all knowing. That is your right and your duty to yourself.

Building your sisterhood circle means making a list and gathering phone numbers for those who will support you along the way. For example, they might be able to organize a "food tree" for after the birth. A food tree is when a circle of support women gather together to bring you meals for the first two weeks after you birth your baby. Your sisters rotate dropping off at least one meal a day, and they organize the drop-off times with you to fit your schedule with the baby. This initial help with the cooking is so valuable and allows you more quality precious time with your newborn.

Your sisterhood circle can als provides childcare during the birth and right after if you have other children and they can go on small errands for you and your family. You may also want to think about who, if anyone, you would like to be present at the birth.

Use these contact pages to fill in the following information about your circle of support. This way, you will have everything you need in one spot when you go into labor.

Frequently Asked Pregnancy Questions

DR. ROBERT BITER, MD

Women should begin the process of finding the right midwife or doctor to care for them during their pregnancy long before making a single appointment. I encourage women and their partners to ask themselves what are their fears, what are the things that they would like to experience differently during the transformation of birth, where do they want to deliver. After becoming clear in their minds, the choice of provider becomes easier.

Here is a quick list of some "good questions" to ask your birthing practitioners:

1. What are their beliefs about birth?

2. Do they have restrictive guidelines regarding birth positions?

3. Can people be present at birth?

4. Do they have rules around the length of second stage laboring or pushing? Will they order a C-Section after a certain amount of pushing time?

5. Why have they dedicated their lives to this work?

6. VERY IMPORTANT: Finally, doctors and midwives will tell you exactly who they are. The key is to listen and believe them.

Natural remedies for morning sickness

The following information is provided by the amazing midwives at The Sanctuary Birth and Wellness Center.

· Himalayan Goji Juice! Mix 8 oz. of goji juice with 1 liter of water and sip throughout the day.

· Eat several small meals throughout the day and try to eat a little before you get hungry. This makes a big difference.

· Avoid greasy foods and foods high in fat content.

- Take 4 or more gelatin caps of powered ginger in the morning and throughout the day if needed.

Important iron-rich foods

If you are iron deficient throughout your pregnancy, try increasing your iron with these foods: (RDA for pregnancy is 30 mg.) Also cook your food in a cast iron pan.

- 1 tablespoon a day of black strap molasses
- raw pumpkin seeds (¼ cup)
- black beans (1 cup cooked)
- almonds (1 cup)
- beef (3 oz)
- millet (¼ cup)
- shrimp (3 oz.)
- raisins (½ cup)
- oatmeal (1 cup / cooked)
- kale (1 cup / cooked)
- wheat germ (¼ cup)

Pregnancy tea recipes

RED RASPBERRY LEAF TEA
1 oz. loose tea combined with 1 quart hot water.
Let steep for 8 hours in the refrigerator. Drink 3–4 cups a day.

OAT STRAW TEA
1 oz. loose tea combined with 1 quart hot water.
Let steep for 4 hours in the refrigerator. Drink 3–4 cups a day.

NETTLES TEA
1 oz. loose tea combined with 1 quart hot water.
Let steep for 4 hours in the refrigerator. Drink 3–4 cups a day.

LAST 6 WEEKS OF PREGNANCY:

FENNEL SEED

1 oz. loose tea combined with 1 quart hot water.
Let steep for 30 minutes. Drink 3–4 cups a day.

BLESSED THISTLE

1 oz. loose tea combined with 1quart hot water.
Let steep for 4 hours. Drink 3–4 cups a day.

LABOR-ADE

Make ahead of time and freeze to use as ice chips or drink the lemonade to restore electrolyte balance and prevent dehydration:

⅓ cup lemon juice
⅓ cup quality local honey
¼ teaspoon sea salt
1 calcium tablet
filtered water to make 1 quart

Mix and blend well.

FOOD TREE ❧

Food Restrictions:

_____

_____

_____

_____

Favorite Foods:

_____

_____

_____

_____

Dates for Delivery:

Breakfast

_____

_____

Lunch

_____

_____

Dinner

_____

_____

Birth Plan Contacts ❧

Contact _____

Phone _____

Email _____

Contact _____

Phone _____

Email _____

Contact _____

Phone _____

Email _____

Contact _____

Phone _____

Email _____

Contact _____

Phone _____

Email _____

Say this as your mantra: *Birth is a natural and normal process.*

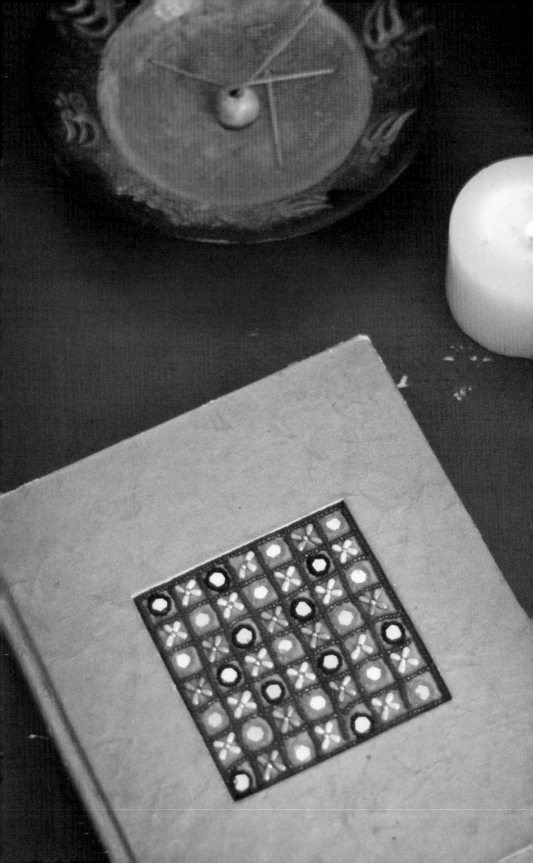

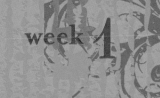

Journal

dive into your story

YOUR BODY ❧

You are on the road to pregnancy—congratulations! If this is a conscious conception, or planned pregnancy, you will already be prepping your body by eating well and opening yourself to what lies ahead. This journey is a roller coaster of emotions and though you are not even technically pregnant during the first week, something IS happening in your body, and luckily your body knows just what to do to prepare itself for this journey. Your egg is still on its path to fertilization and because your due date is calculated by using the first day of your last period, this first week is not yet a pregnancy. However, the lining of your uterus is preparing itself for a potential pregnancy by thickening.

YOUR BABY ❧

During this first week, you're not technically pregnant yet. Weird, huh? This is actually the week of your menstrual period and your egg has dropped and is trying to get fertilized. Think of it this way, during these early days, your baby is basically just knocking at the door of your uterus, wanting to be invited in, to get settled, and hang out for a while. While you are getting ready to be pregnant, it is never too early to begin taking prenatal vitamins, eating healthily, and exercising.

YOUR SPIRIT ❧

Bringing a baby into the world is a big deal! It requires planning and thoughtful emotional processing. When you begin this journey of wanting to have a baby, prepare to be pushed and stretched to all of your limits. Know that you are strong enough to handle it all, but go into it aware and full of confidence. This is the very beginning of a long road, so try to remind yourself that this truly is a journey and not a destination. Once this baby starts growing in your body, you are a mother for the rest of your life. Allow yourself the necessary time to prepare for the path ahead by implementing both physical and spiritual practices that will help you and your baby thrive.

WEEK 1 ℮⁓

Journaling is a great way to explore your personal journey of pregnancy. Getting pregnant is a blessed and joyous event, but there are many other feelings that can and do arise throughout the process. If you are able to get a journaling practice started early on, you may find it a very helpful tool through all the twists and turns you are likely to experience. Give yourself the gift of journaling and become the scribe of your life, noting the important milestones that you cross as you grow this baby into being.

Reflections

Once you have made the decision to try to get pregnant and have a baby, start the emotional prep work. This is a great time, before the baby arrives, to really look closely at why you want to have a child, what kind of parenting philosophy you have and whether it matches your partner's, what your hopes and dreams are for this pregnancy, and what you envision your birth looking like. These are huge questions and take some time to answer, so starting this internal dialogue now will better help guide you down this path as you get deeper into it. Use the journal pages in this book as a space to record your thoughts, plans, and desires.

Ideas

· Help your baby get a fresh start by cutting out caffeine, alcohol, and smoking (if you do). Eat foods high in folic acid and begin taking prenatal vitamins. Try New Chapter organic vitamins, as they are whole-food based probiotic vitamins that support you and fetal development.

· Create a journal practice for yourself. Take a few moments every morning to write down your intentions for the day and a few moments in the evening to close out your day with your thoughts and feelings. This structured way of journaling will become a valuable tool and second nature after some time and will organically help you deal with your feelings as they arise.

Website Pairing

Conscious Conception and Pregnancy
  http://www.consciousconceptionandpregnancy.com/index.html

Book Pairing

Conscious Conception by Jeannine Parvati Baker and Frederick Baker
The True and the Questions by Sabrina Ward Harrison

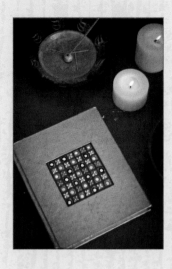

Journaling

Take a few moments to describe your process of conception and journal about your walk down the road to a sacred pregnancy.

dive into your story

Journaling

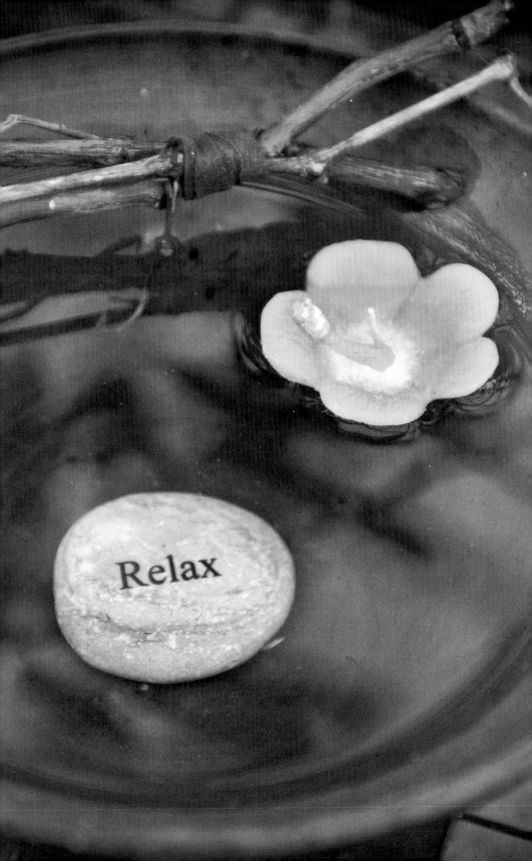

Sacred Space

claim your space

YOUR BODY ⓔ◟

Your body is a temple, a sacred space, and will create and house the most precious being in the world, your child. Your body is just getting warmed up to the idea that a living, growing being will be inside you and needs to start working hard to create the necessary space for your baby to grow. Being busy women, who rarely slow down, we sometimes need our bodies to take over and ensure that we get the rest we need, which is why you are feeling tired and run down. Listen to your body and rest! This is Mother Nature's way of helping women honor and respect the process of creating a human being.

YOUR BABY ⓔ◟

During this second week of this process, funny enough, you are still not technically pregnant. The egg is on its way to fertilization, and likely will be set at the end of this week, and although you will have to wait to find out whether you are having a boy or a girl, the gender is already determined at this early stage.

YOUR SPIRIT ⓔ◟

Women who enter into pregnancy and motherhood are brave and carry the collective energy of all those women who came before them and birthed babies—and themselves in the process. As you prepare you spirit for the road ahead, know your strength, know your power, and know that you and this baby were meant to be together. Everything is perfect, no matter what your circumstances, and you and your baby will grow together and discover each day as it passes.

WEEK 2 ⌁

Every woman needs a special spot to call her own, a sacred space where she can keep special items close to her heart, an altar that reflects her life in any given moment. At the beginning of this pregnancy process, create a special spot in your home as a constant reminder of how amazing this road is, so that every time you see this space or take the time to sit in front of it and light a candle, you will immediately be reminded of how valuable what you are doing truly is. You are creating life and being conscious about your choices. We all lose our way from time to time and this sacred spot will help keep you on track. This book presents a series of projects for creating sacred objects to place on your altar to empower and ready yourself for birth. By the end of this process, your "pregnancy power altar" should be filled with your birth art, mantras, pictures, candles, and other important things you may pick up along the way.

Reflections

Having a space that you claim as your own is a constant reminder to slow down, even if for only a moment every day. This practice will help to bring your pregnancy into your spiritual awareness, rather than only focusing on your physical being, which is far easier to do. Remember that this space is JUST for you, and should be respected as such by others in the home. You may want to transition this space to a family altar at some point after the arrival of your baby. Take your time creating this space and make sure it really reflects this experience for you. When you do sit in front of it, light a candle and try to envision holding your baby in your arms and remind yourself how powerful you are.

Ideas

- Choose a spot in your home that is both comfortable and inspiring to you. Make it pretty! You want to spend time in your space, so keep things like fresh flowers, your birth art, this book, your pregnancy calendar, candles, incense, sage, oils, a pregnant goddess figurine, and any other special items that represent this pregnancy to you. Perhaps keep a pillow in front of the space so you will be able to sit with ease.

- Take a moment each day to sit in front of the altar and say hello to your baby.
- When you go into labor take something from your altar to use as a focal point and a reminder of your strength as a mother.

Inspirational Card Pairing

Try having some motivational or inspirational cards at the altar and pull one out every time you sit in front of the altar to deepen your personal practice. Try the *Self-Care Cards* by Cheryl Richardson.

Music Pairing

Choose some peaceful relaxing music to play while you sit at your altar. Try *The Book of Secrets* album by Loreena McKennitt or Donna DeLory's *The Lover and the Beloved*.

Candle Pairing

Pure Light Candles
  www.cleannaturalhealty.com

Book Pairing

The Smudging and Blessing Book by Jane Alexander

journal on

Sacred Space

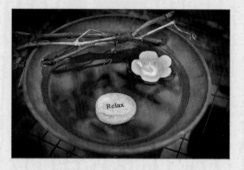

Take a picture of your special space and tape it into this book. Write about the process of setting up this space and what significance the individual items have to you.

claim your space

journal on

Sacred Space

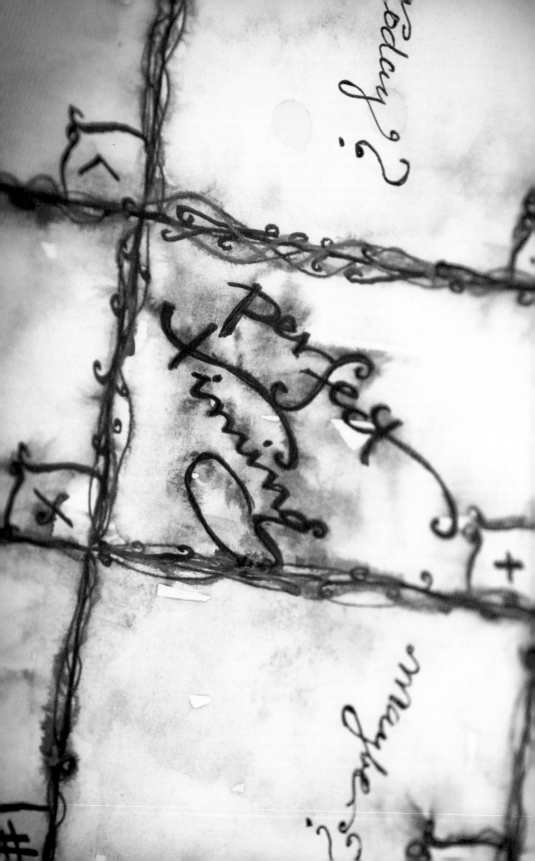

Due date

*your baby knows
the right day to come*

trust the process

YOUR BODY ⸂⸌

You are finally pregnant—congratulations!

Remember that your due date is typically calculated by the first day of your last menstrual period. Every pregnancy is unique and your body will respond to this journey differently every time. Right now what is most important is diet. Make sure you are eating proteins, which will help the baby create new tissue, and extra iron like from leafy greens, red meat, eggs, and legumes (you should also cook in cast iron pans during pregnancy). The baby needs a lot of iron to create extra blood, dairy and calcium products for growing bones, and lots of water! The pregnancy hormones will start kicking in and you will start feeling tired, so beginning to nurture yourself with good whole foods will help you feel better too.

YOUR BABY ⸂⸌

During this third week of the pregnancy process, you will have missed your period and will figure out that you are pregnant. The placenta and your baby are starting to form, and although he started as one single cell, he is working overtime to multiply cells like crazy. Your baby has already grown into millions of cells by week three! Can you believe that? When you find out you are pregnant and are informed of your due date, it can help you determine the potential astrological sign of your baby as well, which will help guide you in relating to your baby before he is born.

YOUR SPIRIT ⸂⸌

Finding out you are pregnant is filled with a lot of complexities. Most women feel excited and want to experience those special moments of telling their loved ones the big news, but it can also be filled with a variety of emotions like ambivalence, anxiety, and fear. Having a baby changes your life in major ways, and those changes can bring about so many feelings. No matter what they are, please honor all of the feelings you may have, as that is the most effective tool in dealing with the twists and turns of being pregnant. Use the "due date" as a good guesstimate, but know that your baby will arrive on the perfect day at the perfect time.

WEEK 3 ⌒〰

Figuring out when your baby is "due" is an exciting time. It is filled with a variety of emotions and it's important to acknowledge them all early on. You are likely elated and filled with joy, but you may also be worried, nervous, and somewhat anxious. If this is your first child, these feelings may be around the unknown and if this is not your first baby, your feelings may relate to a whole slew of other issues. Take time in these first days to just let the information marinate while you adjust to the news yourself. Perhaps wait a couple of days before you start to share the information, so that you and your partner can have a few intimate moments with the news before shouting it from the rooftops … which you will inevitably do!

Reflections

Now that you have determined that you are pregnant, really take the time to digest the information and what this baby is going to mean for your life. Let yourself feel all your emotions and take a moment to acknowledge each and every one as if they are good friends stopping by for tea. When you do learn the due date, take the time to figure out what the baby's rising sign will be and start to introduce yourself to him. This relationship will grow and blossom as your body changes to make room for this little guy and it's truly important to really welcome him to your body. This will start the journey off with pure intentions and clarity.

Ideas

· Mark your calendar with the due date you were told, but allow two weeks before that date and two weeks after that date to really be open for possibility. When women say they were "late," all they mean is they went past the date the doctor or midwife told them to expect the child. However, these women were not really late at all. Their births were perfectly timed for when their babies were ready to join the world. So, rather than relying heavily on one day to expect your baby, allow those last weeks to be open and trust your baby and your body to know when and how to birth the baby.

- In addition to keeping this book and journaling what is going on with you, buy a separate calendar just for you and baby to mark important milestones along the way and to keep track of your midwife/doctor appointments. It is a great idea to keep these two books together so they are always with you during these next forty-two weeks. This book and your calendar will become your touchstones during this process and will help you track this journey in many ways.

Book Pairing

Ina May's Guide To Childbirth by Ina May Gaskin
Immaculate Deception II: Myth, Magic and Birth by Suzanne Arms

These are good books to get started with. They will help you learn more about the type of birthing experience you may want to have.

Movie Pairing

The Business of Being Born by Ricki Lake and Abby Epstein

This is a documentary about birthing in America and serves as a great tool to empower women and educate them about all the birthing options available to them.

Food Pairing

Lemon sorbet	Olives
Chamomile and mint teas	Greek yogurt
Ice pops	Kale salads
Nuts	Quinoa
Cheeses	

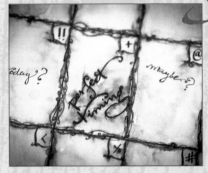

journal on

Your due date

Take a few moments to describe what you felt the moment you found out you were pregnant. What is your due date and what will your child's astrological sign likely be?

your baby knows the right day to come
trust the process

journal on

Your due date

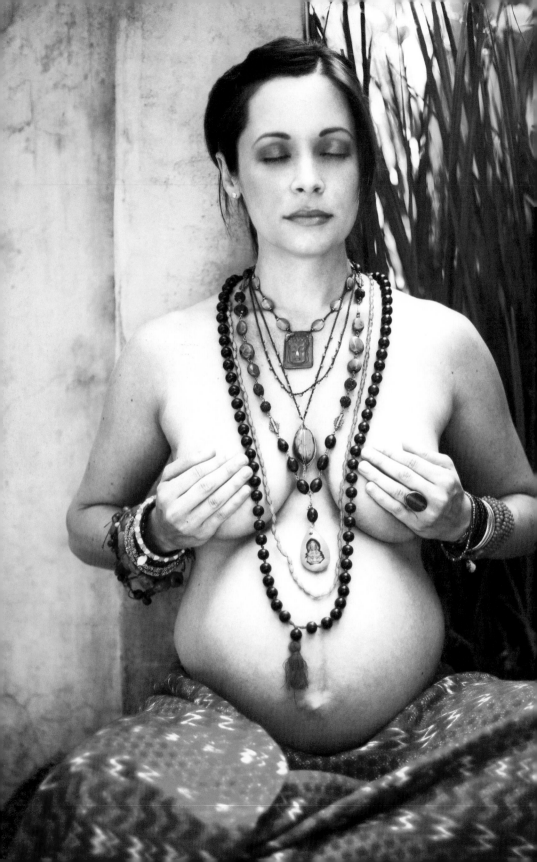

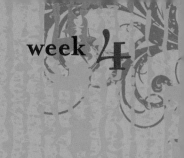

Meditation

breathe deeply

YOUR BODY ☙

During this fourth week of pregnancy, you have essentially just discovered that you are pregnant and although your baby is very small, you can have some big things going on for you physically. You are probably feeling exhausted and a little nauseated and you may have tender breasts. In the pregnant world it's called "morning sickness," although your body clock may not have you feeling funky until the afternoon or evening. One great natural remedy for that is ginger tea or candied ginger. My midwife suggested Himalayan goji juice mixed with a liter of water, to be sipped throughout the day. Goji is also great for headaches and heartburn. The most important thing to remember during this time is to just let your body rest. Deep breathing goes hand in hand with a meditative mind and if you can give yourself the gift of surrender during this time of feeling tired, you will be doing both yourself and the baby a favor. Keep in mind that your body knows how to form a baby and gives you signals of what you need and when. Listen!

YOUR BABY ☙

A baby at four weeks is very small, like a tiny seed, and is starting to settle into your body and make a home within the growing placenta. Although tiny, this little one who will grow into your adorable baby one day. However, at the moment, he most likely resembles a sea creature, but is starting to work hard and fast to develop.

YOUR SPIRIT ☙

You may be going though several emotions at once during this time, and just as it is important for you to allow your body to rest, you must also allow your spirit to rest. Give yourself the space and time you need to let it sink in that you are having a baby. Yes, you are having a baby! Whether this is your first or fourth baby, you need time to introduce yourself to the concept of being pregnant. This time of sleepiness can help provide the emotional space for you to accomplish that. Meditate on your birthing options and decide what is right for you. There are several options including home births, birth-center births, or hospital births. Do your own research and decide what plan works for you, but keep in mind that if you are interested in home or birthing-center options, a midwife can handle all your prenatal care. I would encourage you to think about all the options and talk with professionals in those arenas in order to make the most informed decision possible.

WEEK 4 ⌢

Every medical expert will tell you that lowering your stress levels contributes to a happy and healthy pregnancy. Meditation is an easy way to naturally reduce stress and open yourself to inner peace, but it can be intimidating to many people. However, when you reframe the traditional practice of meditation to look like your everyday life, such as being mindful and present when you do daily tasks like washing dishes or driving, it can become a friendly asset to your pregnancy experience.

Reflections

The deep drink: I was once told by a Buddhist monk that the most important things in our lives are the deep drinks, the moments and experiences we should soak up and enjoy. Growing a baby is the deepest drink from the well of life and even when you are feeling yucky, hold onto that vision.

Slow down your mind, be present with yourself and your growing baby and invite the quiet in. As previously suggested, meditation can take on many forms. It can be sitting in a peaceful place doing deep breathing, or it can be an act of releasing chatter in your mind to maintain conscious presence while engaging in everyday tasks. The important thing to remember when trying to meditate is to make room in your mind for complete awareness in the moment for a sense of calm in your being. This is particularly valuable during pregnancy, as a balanced body, mind, and spirit will encourage an easier physical experience and will give your baby the gift of growing in peace and tranquility. Overall, your stress levels will be lower, which directly impacts the type of pregnancy and birth you have.

Try to maintain a daily practice, even if it's only for five minutes a day. If you can start your day with a few moments of silence, you may see an energy shift in the way your days start to flow. This will benefit both you and your growing baby by reducing your body's stress hormones.

Ideas

- Buy a meditation pillow if you plan on practicing sitting meditation.

- Sit in front of the pregnancy altar you created and ring a bell to signal a quiet time. Then set a timer for however many minutes you have to dedicate to being mindful and present and then ring the bell again when you are finished to signal closure. This is important so that you physically mark your time and space to do this mindfulness practice.

- Buy some nice meditation music that helps you to calm your mind. This can get you in the mood and create an environment that supports the practice. If you do not have time for a daily sitting practice, try playing the music while you engage in other everyday activities to see if it changes your energy.

Book Pairing

The Miracle of Mindfulness by Thich Nhat Hanh or really *anything* by him!

Drink Pairing

Pregnancy support tea
See recipe on page xx.

Music Pairing

Anything by Sheila Chandra, Enya, or Susheela Raman

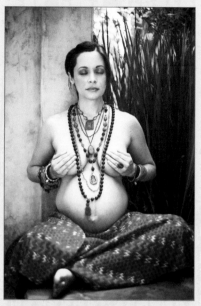

Meditation

Write about what it was like when you took time to stop and really breathe in your surroundings in a more alert state of consciousness. Remember that meditation is not only sitting in front of an altar in silence, but a state of being that allows you to be fully awake in each moment. How can this state of awareness help you to maintain a peaceful pregnancy?

breathe deeply

journal on

Meditation

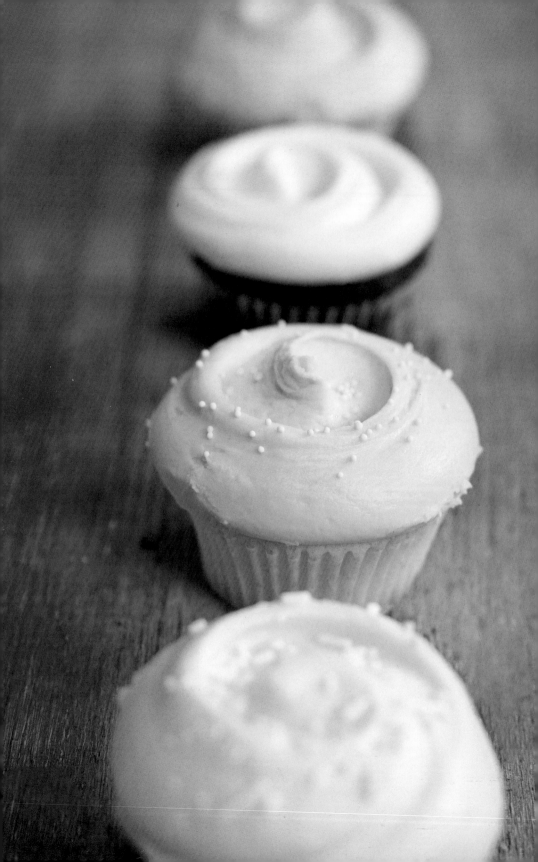

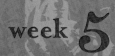

Cravings

dig in … sometimes

YOUR BODY ⟳

During this fifth week, you are undoubtedly tired and feeling all those pregnant symptoms. You may be sick to your stomach one minute and craving pizza and Frosted Flakes the next. Because your hormonal levels are changing at rapid rates, your body responds the best way it can, by forcing you to rest and eat what you need too. Cravings are a mystery, and not everyone experiences them, but you may be surprised by what you start to crave during pregnancy. Hopefully it's kale salad and coconut water, but if you have a craving for a sweet cupcake or cheeseburger, it's okay to indulge a little ... here and there. What is important is maintaining balance between healthy food and any unhealthy cravings. Paying attention to your cravings is also important because it can mean you are deficient in some nutrients. For example, if you crave chocolate, you may need more Vitamin B. If you crave ice chips, you may be deficient in iron. Pay attention to your desires, so you can maintain a healthy pregnancy.

YOUR BABY ⟳

A baby at five weeks is very tiny, and many say he/she resembles a tadpole more than anything else. A healthy little baby growing in your womb is about the size of a bean and your baby's heart, central nervous system, and even bones and muscles will start forming rapidly from this point on. Right around five weeks, your baby also starts forming a skeleton. Although you have already started the process, now is also a good time to decide who you want to catch the baby at birth. Do you want a home birth with a midwife? A birth-center birth with a midwife or a hospital birth with a doctor? Consider those first moments of your baby's life and meditate on what you think will work for you and your family and remember to research your options. Allow room for things to shift and know that the perfect birth is awaiting you. See the Frequently Asked Pregnancy Questions on page xix for some ideas.

YOUR SPIRIT ⌾⌾

Pregnancy is a raw experience. It can open you up in ways you have never imagined and can be both a newfound freedom and a suddenly structured lifestyle. As you settle into your pregnancy physically, so must you accept and embrace where this journey is taking you spiritually. Allow there to be room to flow in and out of various feelings in a way that allows you movement to examine your past, live in the present, and plan for your future. Take time to really examine how often you deny yourself or say no. Practice saying yes to yourself more. Yep, that's right, say YES to *you!*

WEEK 5 ⌾⌾

Because cravings are a mystery, nobody really knows why some women really do like pickles and ice cream during their pregnancies, but what is well known is that a woman's hormones are so out of whack when she gets pregnant that many things sound good to eat that might not have in the past. Be conscious of your preferences and honor yourself by allowing a treat every now and again, and don't worry about your weight! You are supposed to gain weight during pregnancy and honoring that as a part of the process will give you more freedom to say yes to yourself with a balanced consciousness around your choices.

Reflections

What are you craving right now? Think on that and take the time to look deeply at your patterns in allowing yourself to indulge every so often. What is that like for you and what were your messages about saying yes to yourself growing up? Were you encouraged to say yes to your desires or taught that it is selfish to do things just for you? These are questions that are important to ponder during your pregnancy, as this will directly relate to the kind of parent you will become. If there are changes you want to make regarding this issue, now is the time to do a little work on that. You may be the type of person who puts the needs and desires of everyone else before yourself. If this is you, push yourself to put you first during the pregnancy. As a mother, you will always and forever have a little person wanting something from you. Take the time you need to say yes to you, so you can be present enough to say yes with awareness to your child.

Ideas

- If you have an overactive sweet tooth and want to keep more balanced, get creative! Try turning your unhealthy cravings into healthier versions. For example if you die for ice cream, try making a homemade version using raw agave as the sweetener or make iced sorbets. If you love chocolate, try raw dark chocolate that has not been processed. Raw chocolate is super high in antioxidants and is very good for you. Try using coconut sugar to sweeten homemade cookies and cakes.

- If you crave salty foods, try making homemade potato chips with sea salt or kale Parmesan popcorn.

- Practice saying yes to yourself in some way *every day*! Create a mantra that you place on your pregnancy altar that says, "I am growing a baby and I deserve to relax, enjoy the process, and say *yes* to my desires, as long as I am staying healthy and making conscious choices that benefit myself and my baby."

Book Pairing

Practicing Happy by Tim Daulter and *ICE POP JOY* by Anni Daulter
timdaulter@wordpress.com/

Home Movie Night Pairing

Eat, Pray, Love and *Julie & Julia*

Food Pairing

I happen to know someone who makes great healthy doughnuts! If this is a craving of yours, reach out to Rheiana and ask her to ship you a few. They are delicious! (Rheiana is listed under Resources on page 324.)

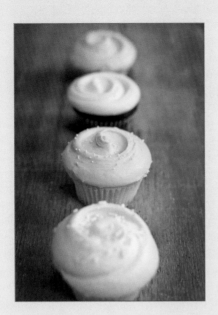

Cravings

What kind of cravings are you
having, if any? Do you have any
great recipes that you have tried
during your pregnancy that you
want again and again?

dig in ... sometimes

journal on

Cravings

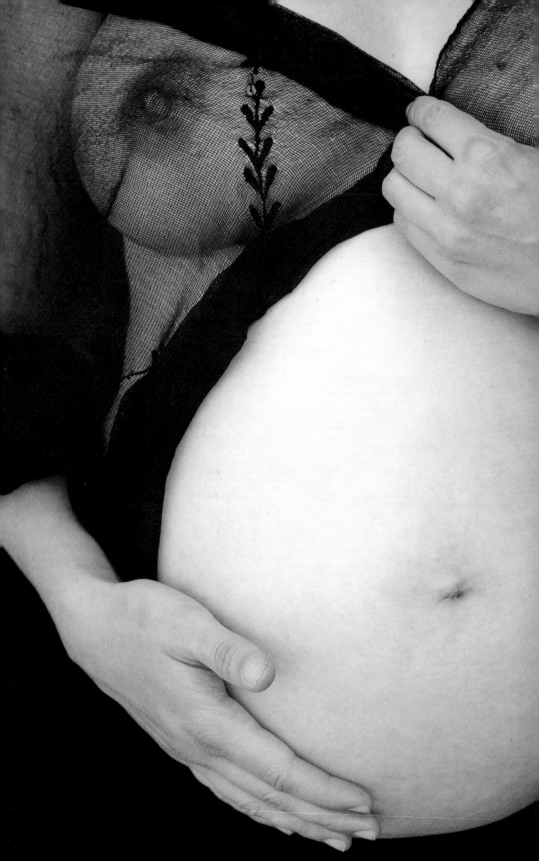

Womb

you create life with your body
and soul with your energy

YOUR BODY ❧

During this sixth week, nausea may be ruling the day and your breasts and nipples will likely be sore and tender. Due to hormonal changes, your breasts are also beginning to grow in preparation for breast-feeding. A tried and true great remedy for sore nipples is Natural Nipple Cream by Earth Mama Angel Baby. Remember that if you are experiencing "morning sickness," try eating *before* you feel hungry. Smaller meals all throughout the day can also help. You may not actually be "showing" yet. But as the symptoms become more and more real, so will your exhale into the pregnancy truly begin.

YOUR BABY ❧

A baby at six weeks is still small, about the size of a little pea, but your body is working hard to circulate blood and form more of the body. Your baby is very busy every moment of the day. At this point, they still resemble a tadpole. Although you can't really hear it yet, your baby's heart is beginning to beat at about the rate of 130 to 150 per minute, about twice what yours does.

YOUR SPIRIT ❧

Your baby is getting get to know you from your womb, and even in these early days, learning happens as you take time to pat your belly or talk with your baby through your womb space. When you are angry or happy your hormones can cross over the placenta, thus affecting your little one's mood as well. Remember that your womb is your baby's home, and your energy feeds your baby's soul. So let your soul shine! Use soothing tones when speaking, and say good morning and good night to your baby every day. Gently speak to her about how wanted and loved she is. Even if science cannot prove that this helps a growing fetus, it sure is a great way to start and end the day!

WEEK 6 ᥠ

Your womb is the center of motherhood. It's the space of protection
for your growing baby and the essence of womanhood. It's the sacred
unknown and within its borders live the mysteries of life itself. A
mother's womb is her most glorious self and deserves deep honoring.
As a woman, you are blessed with the ability to create life, which is an
awesome responsibility. Have reverence for each step of this process
and welcome every changing moment of your pregnancy with your
whole heart. This will impact your energy and your ability to accept
every bump in the road.

Reflections

What have been your thoughts around your womb space before getting pregnant, and how have those thoughts changed now? Keep your
mind clear during your pregnancy, as your thoughts can affect the
energy that you pass along to your baby while she is growing inside
of you. Remember that this womb space is the protection where your
baby feels safe and warm, and she will expect that same comforting feel after entering the world. How will you prepare your womb-
like environment for the baby after birth? In many cultures, mothers
stay inside with their baby for the first month with very few visitors,
just to create the space for bonding time between mother and child.
Think about what is important to you. It's exciting when a new baby is
born and so many people want to come over and visit, but remember
that just because the baby is out of your body, she still needs a warm,
womb-like environment in those beginning days. Try to keep your
visits short and sweet, but without too many distractions. Attention to
these details will ensure a lovely transition into the world.

Ideas

- Try creating some "womb birth art." Make a collage of a circle of
  women's bellies, and put a picture of yours in the center. Notice the
  feelings of protection that you begin to feel as this artwork reframes
  you as the child learning and growing through your pregnancy.

- Honoring time: Take the time to sit in front of your pregnancy altar and honor your womb by thanking it for housing your baby and allowing you to have the experience growing a child within you. Massage in Earth Mama Body Butter (by Earth Mama Angel Baby) all over your belly as you take this honoring time to connect with your womb.

- Create a daily mantra for you to say to your baby, like "You are loved and wanted. I am so excited to meet you very soon."

Music Pairing

"This Woman's Work" by Kate Bush (The version by Maxwell is amazing too.)
Have this playing while you create your art. It's so inspiring.

Drink Pairing

Organic Peaceful Mama Tea by Earth Mama Angel Baby

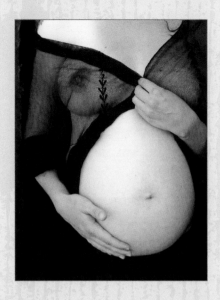

Womb

Write a declaration to protect your child and your relationship with her as she grows. How will you hand down the privilege of being a woman to your daughter and the respect of woman to your son?

you create life with your body and soul with your energy

journal on

Womb

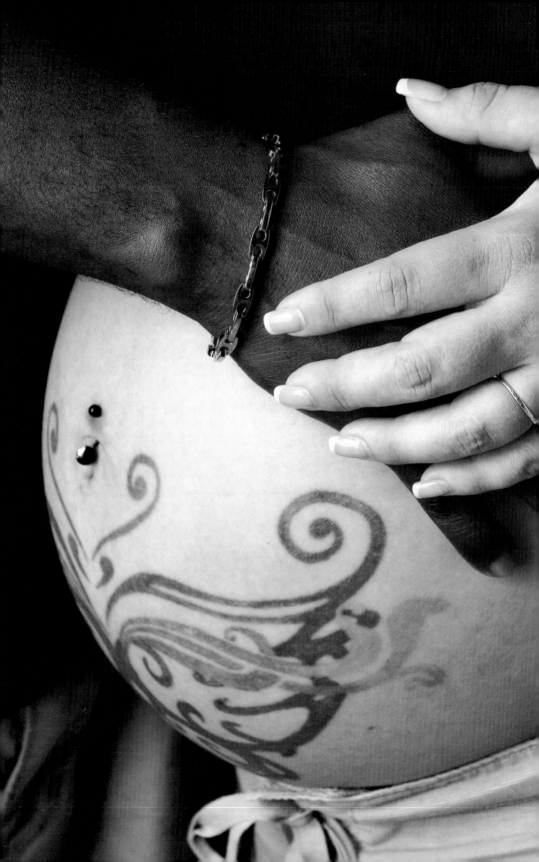

Expectations

every moment,
and every birth experience,
is meant to be …

YOUR BODY ᏋᏕ

You may be getting tired of feeling crappy and run-down. Just know that this comes to an end. For most women, this lasts only through the first trimester. On the other hand, you may not be experiencing anything but pure bliss, and if that is the category you fall into, be grateful and don't ask questions. Just enjoy. Although your uterus has doubled in size by the seventh week and will continue to grow as time passes, you may not even be "showing" yet. Know that you will be able to see that belly bump in no time! Also, if you have not settled on a practitioner by now and are still interviewing, it's time to make your choice. Whether you choose a midwife or an OB-GYN, get connected with those you want to help support you through this process.

YOUR BABY ᏋᏕ

Your baby at seven weeks is now about the size of a small nut. Although she is starting to take more shape, she still has web-like feet and hands and just slight indentations of facial features. What is valuable to remember about you and your baby during this week is that your baby and you are the perfect fit, and are meant to be. This acknowledgment means a lot as you pass through each week, knowing that even if you are uncomfortable or nauseated, you both are meant to experience the other in the exact way you are right now. Be grateful and love your body and your baby for who they are in this moment.

YOUR SPIRIT ᏋᏕ

As you gear up for all that awaits you, both in the pregnancy and during the birthing process, be acutely aware of what you "expect" to happen. None of these expectations may be based in any sort of reality, but may stem from what you have heard from others, what you have seen happen with friends, or things you have read in magazines or books. Try to separate your own experience from that of others, as each pregnancy is unique. Although there are of course similarities, no pregnancy is ever the same as another (even your own multiple pregnancies will be different). This is important to remember as you gear up for the journey ahead. Staying flexible and moving through your pregnancy with confidence are the keys to a successful experience, even if the outcomes end up somewhat different than you expect. Take time to talk through your pregnancy and birth expectations with your partner and birthing support team.

WEEK 7 ⌒

Energy flows where attention goes.
—MICHAEL BECKWITH

Most people have certain expectations when it comes to being pregnant, having a baby, and then raising him. We all have visions or fantasies about what it will be like and that becomes our expectations. The danger of having such expectations is that if and when things do not turn out as we may have planned, we can become depressed, angry, and frustrated with our lives. However, when we walk more in the flow of the universe and our lives, the path that has unexpected and perhaps unwanted twists becomes exciting. When we own and embrace that approach, we look forward to the "not knowing" and are excited about the many gifts life hands us.

Reflections

What expectations do you have for this pregnancy? What expectations do you have for your baby and yourself as a mother? These are very important questions to begin to ask yourself as you move through this reflective period. Be honest with yourself. You are not a "bad" mother if you expect that your pregnancy will be easy, the birth will be effortless, and your baby will never shed a tear. What is important is just to acknowledge what your expectations are now. If you are meant to experience slight variations or drastic differences from those expectations, you can be in your own flow. You can accept what comes with grace and the knowledge that this path belongs only to you and your baby, and is cherished for that simple reason alone.

Ideas

- Meditate on where you gather your ideas from and all the messages you have been given about what your pregnancy and motherhood is "supposed" to be like. Just make a mental note.

- Acceptance rock art project: Find a beautiful rock that has a nice flat surface. Paint the word "Acceptance" on it and decorate it how you like. This will serve as a physical reminder to be in the flow of your life and to offer an open invitation to what is meant to come without resistance or fear. Keep this special rock on your pregnancy altar and even have it present at the birth. This could be used a focal point during your surges.

- Talk with your midwife and or OB-GYN about any feelings you are having relating to how the pregnancy is going for you in an emotional way. It may help to hear her or his perspective.

Book Pairing

Zen Ties by Jon J. Muth and David Pittu and *The Boy Who Ran into the Woods* by Jim Harrison

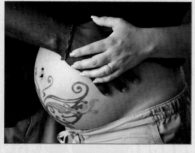

Expectations

May we be safe.
May we happy.
May we have good health
And enough to eat,
And may we live at ease of heart
With whatever comes to us in life.

—*Metta Meditation by* KRISHNA DAS

Make a list of your expectations around this pregnancy. Where did you get those messages and how can you prepare yourself to be open for what is meant to come?

every moment, and every birth experience, is meant to be ...

journal on

Expectations

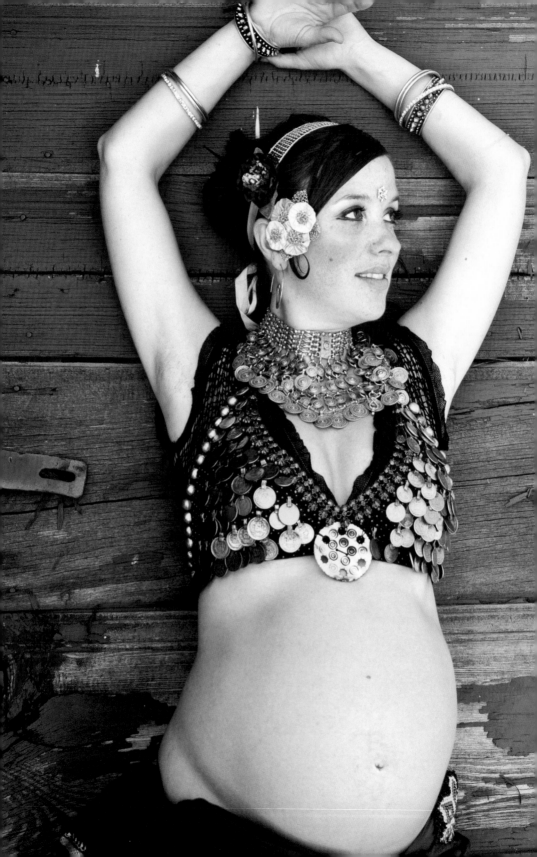

Body Image

love your new curves

YOUR BODY ☙

Your body is definitely feeling pregnant and you may even have a little bump now. So it's time to really start noticing how you feel as your body changes along with your growing baby. You may still be feeling a little ill and you might be sensitive to certain smells and foods. If you are nauseated and are not eating food, make sure you are taking your prenatal vitamins to supplement what you may not be getting. I like New Chapter prenatal vitamins, as they are whole-food based and organic. It's also perfectly normal for you to feel light cramping as your uterus is expanding, but any bleeding should be reported to your midwife or doctor. You might be getting over being so exhausted now and having a tiny bit more energy. So even though your favorite jeans might be getting tight, you are just starting to wake up to the reality of pregnancy now. Your introductions are done and your body is settling in.

YOUR BABY ☙

A baby at eight weeks is starting to take on a more human shape and is developing eyelids, ears, fingers, and toes and is about the size of a blackberry (the fruit, not the phone). The body is starting to expand a little bit to make more room for forming organs and you can just see the forming of a little nose now!

YOUR SPIRIT ☙

You may be both excited and frustrated. Having completed the first three months of your pregnancy while nurturing yourself and your baby through the beginning weeks of life will bring you a sense of accomplishment. Remember that this is also an exciting time as you are finally able to see your little belly bump. Keep in mind that those tight jeans are a sign of a healthy baby to come.

WEEK 8 ⌒

When a woman gets pregnant, she goes through many emotional and physical changes. The most obvious change is her growing belly and the reshaping of her body to accommodate a new being. For many women, gaining weight is associated with being unattractive and does not match her societal consciousness of what is acceptable. The media and print magazines tend to dictate what is, and what is not, beautiful, and many women have their self-image tied primarily to their body image.

Growing a baby means gaining weight. Pure and simple, your baby needs you to gain weight in order to blossom into a healthy newborn. The question is how you feel about this new body of yours and how it relates to your self-image.

Reflections

Take some time to honor your new body as it blossoms into a mother's body: one that will produce milk to nourish your baby, one that will expand to let your baby enter into the world, and one that will need mothering hips to carry your baby when she needs to be close. Meditate on all of your feelings that arise in relation to gaining weight and having a newly developed body. Ask yourself if you feel sexy and attractive or if you have feelings of being undesirable and ugly. Take notice of all of your feelings and acknowledge them, have compassion with yourself and own them. We are perfect in every moment. Remember that your new curves are luscious and full of life.

Ideas

- Stand naked in front of a mirror and let your belly be full and glorious and see what feelings it brings up in you.

- Wear something that makes you feel sexy and gorgeous that accentuates your new body.

- Have your big belly decorated with a lovely henna design to honor its beauty.

- Have a pregnancy photo shoot to document and show off all of your new curves!

Food Pairing

Go out for your favorite meal to celebrate the completion of the first two months of your pregnancy.

Book Pairing

A Woman's Worth by Marianne Williamson

Website Pairing

Proud Body (belly casting and paints)
www.proudbody.com

Fun Outing Pairing

A trip to the organic Day Spa! Try Arborederm if you are in LA (the owner is amazing and specializes in pregnant mamas!), and if not, try to locate one in your area.
www.arborederm.com

Body Image

How do you feel about your new growing belly and gaining weight? What
messages have you been taught about
this? Take time to journal about how
you see yourself as your baby is growing inside of you.

love your new curves

journal on
Body Image

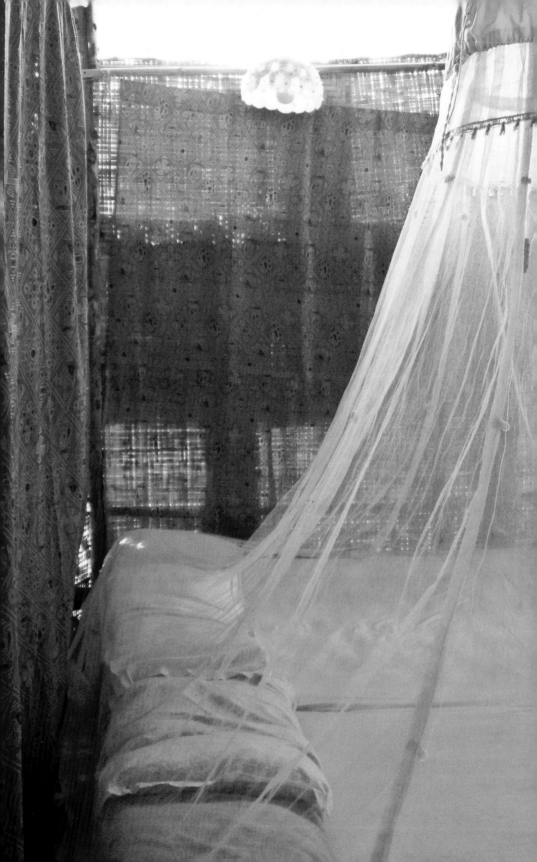

Romance

celebrate intimacy

YOUR BODY ☙

What was your body like before you were pregnant? Can you even remember now? Oftentimes, it feels like the baby owns your body and you are merely a visitor. As your belly bump grows, so are your feelings about how your "look" is changing. By the ninth week you may not feel like being romantic or opening up that well of connection as you are likely still trying to cope with getting acclimated to your pregnancy. Know that your body needs to be touched and held through this process. Keep your stress levels down using physical touch from your partner, and this will reduce some common symptoms of early pregnancy like headaches and anxiety.

YOUR BABY ☙

Your baby at nine weeks is around one inch long and is starting look more human. Your baby wants you and your partner to maintain a healthy relationship, as this will ultimately reduce your stress and allow for a more healthy pregnancy, so make sure to nurture the baby by caring for your relationship. Although for most people it is okay to have sex throughout your entire pregnancy and will not harm the baby, check with your practitioner if you have special situations in which you are concerned about it. Your baby's sex organs are likely formed by now, but you will not be able to determine if you are having a boy or a girl until about thirteen weeks or after.

YOUR SPIRIT ☙

Your hormones are raging. As a result, you may be feeling quite moody and not particularly romantic, but staying connected to your partner during this process is critical. Honor the fact that the two of you created this little life growing inside of you and that this baby came from the love that you share for one another. Create the space to really spend quality time with your lover and share this experience with him or her. Remember that your partner wants to be included in this process, so the more you can share with each other, the stronger your relationship will stay as you hit rough patches.

WEEK 9 𝒢

Your relationship with your partner is shifting and will continue to change as time passes and the focus becomes all about the baby. Take the time you have now to enjoy each other, nurture your relationship by spending time together, and keep the communication open as your relationship deepens throughout this process. It is very easy to make everything about the baby, but this time is also about the two of you and that cannot be moved to the back burner. Keep your relationship fresh with excitement as you share this journey together.

Reflections

Was this a planned, conscious pregnancy or a surprise? How has the news affected your relationship with your partner? Have you noticed any differences and has it brought you closer together? Make sure to keep talking throughout this process! Talk about everything as it is happening. Make sure to include your partner in how you are feeling, both physically and emotionally. Remember that even though your partner is not pregnant, he or she may also be feeling symptoms right along with you. This is one of the mysteries of relationships during pregnancy, but the feelings are real and should not be ignored. You are the star of this show for sure, but your partner has a leading role, and needs to be included in what is going on with you. A baby will end up right between the two of you almost every night, so make sure to take time now to appreciate each other and to lay the foundation for a healthy relationship after baby comes.

Ideas

- Dates: Go out at least once a week with your partner. Dinner and a movie, walks on the beach, picnics in the park, yoga on Saturday mornings followed by a nice big breakfast, a day spent at home in bed eating favorite foods and reading together, or just a simple shared bath with essentials oils—these are all great ideas to keep connected and enjoy each other as you both walk this path.

- Ask your partner to give you a massage and end it with a lovemaking session.

- Keep the dialogue open at all times, as this process should be a shared journey and not an isolated one.

Home Movie Pairing

The Notebook

Before Sunrise

Shakespeare in Love

Like Water for Chocolate

Music Pairing

"You are Amazing" by Josh Kelly

"Just Want You Around" by Lauryn Hill

"These Arms of Mine" by Otis Redding

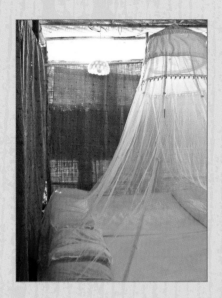

Romance

What is the romantic connection
between you and partner now that
you are pregnant? Is there any
difference? What would you like
to be different and how can you
encourage more romance between
you?

celebrate intimacy

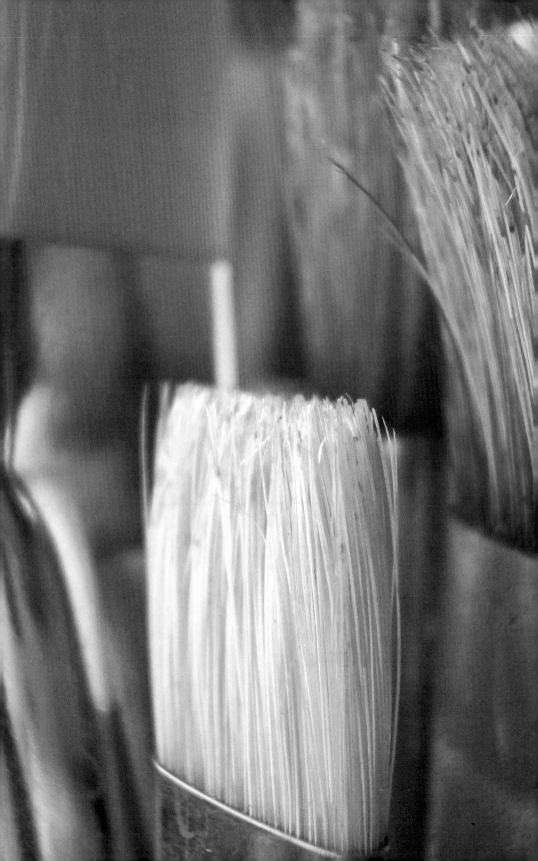

Birth Art Expression

design your birth experience

YOUR BODY ⟡⟋

You may begin to feel some constipation during this week. It is totally normal. Some natural remedies: increase your fiber and eat more whole grains like millet, quinoa, pasta, and breads. Raw fruits, especially kiwis and prunes, and raw veggies are good choices too. Really anything high in fiber will help with that. As this is a week to really focus on being creative, see what fun recipes you can create that may help with the constipation and any morning sickness you may be experiencing. Whatever you do, don't skip meals! Try to eat small portions BEFORE you feel sick, and that will help calm your stomach and give you a little energy. I know there may be times when you may not want to eat at all, but remember that this is the fuel that your baby needs to grow into your arms, so when you eat, make it count.

YOUR BABY ⟡⟋

A baby at ten weeks is about the size of a strawberry (about an inch long) and is really beginning to form some bodily features. The critical development phase is over and now it is time for rapid development to take place. Your baby is forming fingernails now and vital organs are creating lots of red blood cells. The baby can kick around and is now forming little elbows. And all of the baby's limbs can bend! Cool! Draw a symbol, like a waterfall or an om sign or any other symbol that represents this journey for you, to represent your baby growing through this first trimester.

YOUR SPIRIT ⟡⟋

Being forced by your body to slow down leaves you with more time to spiritually connect with yourself and your growing baby. You may not consider yourself a creative person, but keep in mind you are the ultimate creatrix—you are making a person! That is an incredible miracle and your baby is as perfect as you are and only *you* can create *your* baby. Give yourself the time you need to begin to see the mother in you emerge.

WEEK 10 ⌒

There are many ways to enjoy a sacred pregnancy, and one of them is by making birth art. This is a special form of art that is connected to your pregnancy and this particular baby. No matter how many children you have, each one is unique and your birth art creation should reflect that.

Reflections

Take some time in the next day or so to think about how you can make your pregnancy more sacred through some type of artistic expression. This could be painting a picture, making a collage, or using clay to mold a figure of courage that can be with you at the birth (or any other form that feels right to you). Birth art is unique to you and your experience as you bond with your baby who is growing inside of you. How you express this through art can be transformative and healing.

This project can be done alone or with your partner. It is nice to include your partner if she or he is willing to participate, as it can help to build the closeness between your partner and your baby. In addition, it can be an opportunity for you both to enjoy something fun together that can also serve as a heartfelt gift to your baby later on in his life.

Please note that this is not an exercise in how talented you are as an artist. Free expression through art is just an opportunity for you to use other means to enjoy your pregnancy. As you are a vessel of creation for your baby, try to befriend your inner artist, and bring to life a piece of birth art, or several, that is a true expression of your experience with this pregnancy in the here and now.

Ideas

- Buy a set of watercolor paints and paper and free form paint by choosing colors that really speak to you. Paint a picture for yourself that relates to this pregnancy.

- Get old magazines and cut out images or words that express what you are feeling about becoming a mother. Develop a "collage of inspiration" for yourself and have it present at the birth.

- Buy some beads and create a special necklace for yourself that you can wear at the birth. This birth empowerment necklace should be weaved with intention and when you are beading it, say a mantra such as, "I am strong and join with all women who have birthed before me and I will birth this baby easily!"

Music Pairing

Bon Iver!
I love this guy. Listen to the song "Skinny Love."
Anything by Ray LaMontagne

Website Pairing

Dirty Footprints Studio
www.dirtyfootprints-studio.com
Playtime with Your Inner Muse
www.shop.artizencoaching.com
Tamara Laporte (willowing)
www.willowing.com

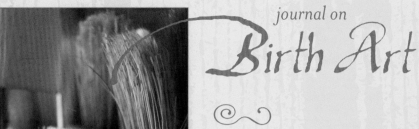

journal on

Birth Art

Name your art piece. There is power in calling something that you have birthed by its own name. Take some time to journal about your experience with forming your birth art and maybe use this space to draw a sketch of it!

design your birth experience

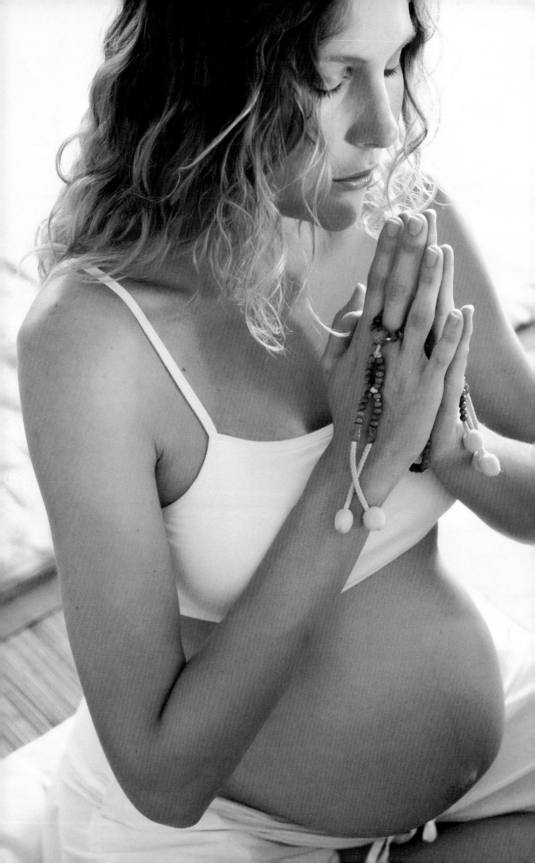

Exercise

stay strong for birthing

YOUR BODY ⌒

Growing a baby means a lot of work for your body and regular exercise can help reduce the various aches and pains of pregnancy. At around eleven weeks, you might start having "round ligament" pains around your abdomen, as your body stretches and makes room for your baby. Regular stretching, and especially prenatal yoga, could help with this tremendously. A regular routine will also help you get more sleep, reduce pregnancy headaches, and prepare you physically for birthing your baby. It is also great to get into a daily rhythm of doing Kegel exercises. These are the contracting and releasing of the pelvic floor muscles. My midwife would ask me every time I saw her if I had been doing my Kegels and even had stickers made up to place around the house to remind me to "do Kegels." Remember that when you start having surges, when you are in labor, it's super tiring and you need a lot of stamina and physical strength to move that baby out of you and into the world. It's never too late to start getting in shape for the big day!

YOUR BABY ⌒

At eleven weeks, your little cutie finally looks like a little baby, and not an alien you would not recognize. Finger and toenails are forming and your baby, although small, also works out everyday. Your baby rolls around, stretches, and essentially plays to get himself strong for the work he must do to enter the world. You see, the two of you MUST work together come that magical day, so he also needs to be strong and healthy and free of stress in order to peacefully enter the world.

YOUR SPIRIT ⌒

Spiritually you should be settling into being pregnant, and although your pre-pregnancy days are becoming a distant memory, it's important to maintain a "spiritual workout" as well. This would include:

A daily mantra, starting now, that reaffirms that you are strong enough and brave enough to birth your baby. Keep it simple, short and affirming!

Keep communication lines open with your partner at all times, letting him or her know how you are feeling and what you may be struggling with.

Work through the journal pages of this book in a genuine attempt to work through any issues you may have around your own childhood, this pregnancy, or becoming a mother.

Do not hold onto negative feelings or thoughts, as these can affect your baby and your stress levels. Try not to engage in too many arguments or fights with your partner, as the tension will only add to any pregnancy ailments you may be experiencing. Maintaining positive interactions with people reduces physical pains and infuses your pregnancy with joy.

WEEK 11 ⌒◡

Your body needs to be strong and healthy to birth a baby, plain and simple, and carrying a baby around in your body is tiring! Not only are your hormones all over the place, you are charged with the task of eating a lot, sleeping a lot, and keeping yourself healthy. Introducing a regular exercise routine is important, both to keep you feeling fit and boost your energy, but to keep your body strong as you prepare to birth your baby. Yoga is a great way to stay toned, both physically and spiritually, and can be a lovely way to connect with other pregnant mamas to swap pregnancy stories and gain that sisterhood support. Exercise releases natural endorphins in your brain, much like what happens while birthing a baby, and gives you extra energy when you need it.

Reflections

What is your relationship to exercise? Do you have a regular practice? Are you willing to start one now? A prenatal exercise practice should be done with purpose and with the intention to create a strong birthing body. Keep your baby in your thoughts as you prepare your body to bring him into the world.

Ideas

- Look up your local yoga centers to see if they have a prenatal class you can attend.

- Take long walks in the park, around your neighborhood or at the beach. This will help bring down the baby later and help jump start labor at the end of your pregnancy.

Video Pairing

The Divine Mother Prenatal Yoga Series with Anna Getty

Prenatal Yoga with Shiva Rea

Book Pairing

Bountiful, Beautiful, Blissful: Experience the Natural Power of Pregnancy and Birth with Kundalini Yoga and Meditation by Gurmukh Kaur Khalsa

Fitness Pairing

Cindy Crawford's *A New Dimension* DVD
with Kathy Kaehler

Yoga with Jessica Jennings of MaYoga at BINI.
She teaches twice a week and teaches pre- and postnatal yoga around LA. Or find a studio in your area that has prenatal yoga classes.
mayoga.com

Blooma (yoga/wellness education)
www.blooma.com

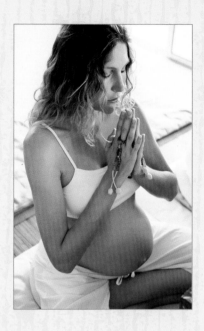

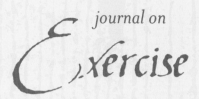

journal on

What is your exercise routine? How is it impacting your moods and feelings of exhaustion?

stay strong for birthing

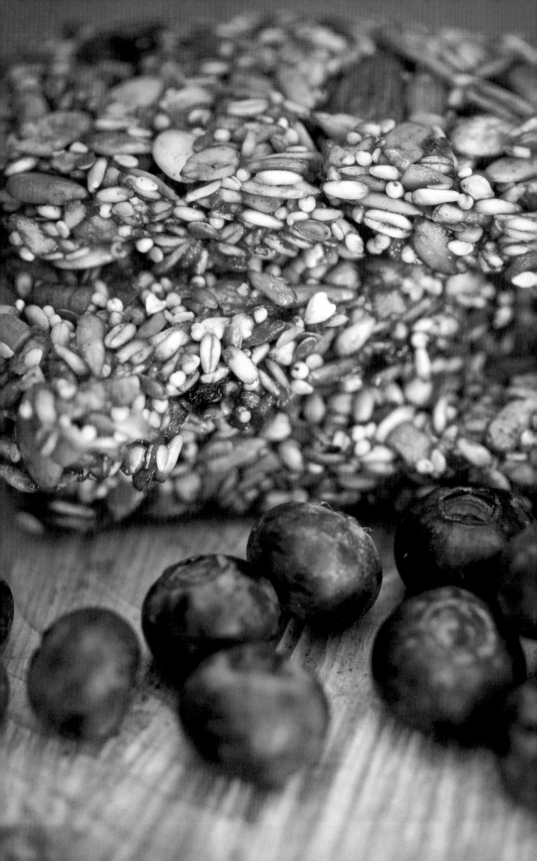

Mindful Eating

*nourish your body, mind,
and soul with mantras
and whole foods*

YOUR BODY ❧

Your belly bump is showing, you are hungry all the time, and your hormones are still a little out of sorts. Good foods to feed your body and jumpstart your mindful eating practice include whole, fresh, organic foods that have been minimally processed, such as salads, whole-grain breads, and soups. Herbal teas, veggie- and fruit-packed smoothies, organic proteins, and of course supergreens like kale are always excellent baby-growing foods. A well-nourished mama is a well-fed baby!

YOUR BABY ❧

Your baby at twelve weeks is hungry too, as she is working hard to grow and gain weight and her umbilical cord is fully formed now. Remember that everything you eat, your baby eats too, so bringing mindful eating and healthy foods into your kitchen is an essential part of creating a strong and vibrant baby. Your little sweetie looks like a baby now, and with a fully developed brain, is starting to act like one too with early stages of yawning and sucking starting to kick in.

YOUR SPIRIT ❧

The first trimester is completed after this week—congratulations! In celebration of the tail end of the first three months and hopefully the end of any nausea, rejuvenate your body and mind and spirit with a trip to your favorite restaurant for a lovely meal to sooth your soul. Food memories are strong in life, and it's a good practice to notice them and honor them. Some foods are comforting, some bring back amazing memories of your own mother or father in the kitchen cooking for you, and some may have heavy strings attached if you have struggled with eating to meet emotional needs. This is a great time to look deeply into what food traditions were passed down to you so that you may make conscious adjustments if needed.

WEEK 12 ⓔ◞

The practice of mindful eating stretches far beyond your pregnancy and hopefully started way before. It is the spiritual practice of conscious cooking and eating, when intention is put into your cooking. Knowing where your food was sourced from is a priority. If you are not a "foodie," it can be overwhelming, but just keep it simple and delicious. If you get into a meditative practice that includes bringing awareness to the kitchen, like saying a verse or a mantra before cooking, this will become second nature when you begin that very critical road of preparing solid foods for your baby.

Reflections

What has your relationship with food been like throughout your life, both before and after being pregnant? Have you spent time finding out what the best foods are and what you should avoid during your pregnancy? With every bite you take, you feed your baby, and your little one is already forming preferences for certain types of foods based on what you eat. Further, the moment you start breast-feeding the baby essentially eats and drinks what you do. Therefore, this is a great time to examine deeply any food issues you may have, as you want to have this stuff worked out and clear before you start introducing solid foods to your baby between the age of seven to eleven months.

What kinds of foods did you eat growing up and what was the "food philosophy" in your home? Create patterns now that you want to pass along to your child. If you have not eaten particularly healthy food in your life, it's never too late to start! Do you eat local? One way to ensure fresh organic foods in your fridge is to buy locally from either a farmer (at the farmers' market), a co-op or even a local CSA (community-shared agriculture). You may consider making your kitchen a sacred space where no fighting or arguing is allowed, thus keeping your food protected from any negative vibes floating around the house. Introducing mindful eating into your life is not only a good practice for pregnant women, it's an amazing way to raise your family. Food awareness and healthy choices are traditions worth handing down.

Ideas

· Create an altar in your kitchen with pictures of your family, a candle, and maybe your favorite blessing. Consider even ringing a mindfulness bell before cooking, when sitting down to eat, and relaxing after you have finished your meal.

· After you have your baby, remember that family mealtime can be a special way to connect with your children.

Book Pairing

The Organic Family Cookbook by Anni Daulter

It's a great family cookbook and will give you a lot of great ideas on healthy choices to make for yourself and your family.

Food Pairing

MY NURTURING ROASTED TOMATO SOUP AND RUSTIC GARLIC BREAD

Ingredients

8 large beef tomatoes	I teaspoon oregano
I whole head of garlic, roasted	I container vegetable stock
I tablespoon olive oil	(16 oz.)
I teaspoon sea salt	2 vegetable bouillon cubes
I teaspoon cracked pepper	I handful kale, chopped
I teaspoon tarragon for tomatoes and I teaspoon for soup	I teaspoon pepper flakes
	I lime
I pat of butter	4 slices of your favorite rustic
I large yellow onion, chopped	bread, turned into toasted garlic bread

Directions

Preheat oven to 350°.

Cut all tomatoes in half and place on a large baking sheet lined with parchment paper. Cut top off garlic head and get all cloves out.

Sprinkle tomatoes with olive oil, salt, pepper, and tarragon.

Add garlic cloves all over the sheet to roast both together.

Roast tomatoes and garlic for 45 minutes.

Add butter to a large soup pot. Add in chopped onion, along with I teaspoon of tarragon and oregano. Brown the onions.

Add in roasted tomatoes and garlic, vegetable stock, bouillon cubes, kale, and red pepper flakes.

Blend the soup together in a blender.

Serve immediately with a wedge of lime to squeeze on top of soup right before eating and garlic bread to dip.

Website Pairing

Food Practice
  www.foodpractice.com

Motherbees (amazing food delivery)
  www.motherbees.com/

journal on

Mindful Eating

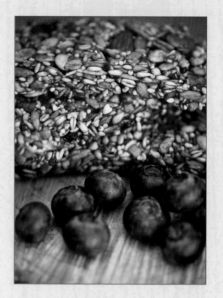

What are your favorite recipes
and foods that you are enjoying
throughout your pregnancy that
you may be able to pass down to
your own child someday?

nourish your body, mind, and soul with mantras and whole foods

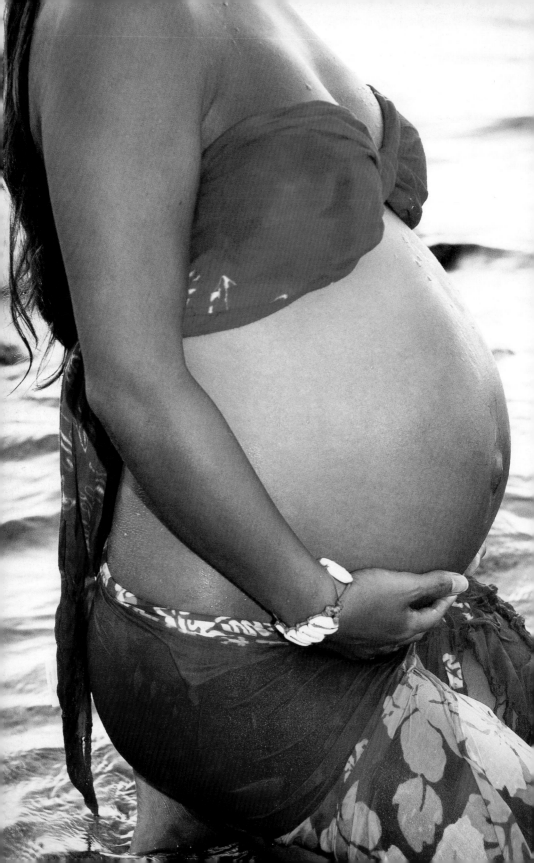

Radiant Glow

hold your belly in gratitude

YOUR BODY ❧

Your body has just accomplished something amazing! It has supported you through your first trimester and has loved and nurtured your baby through the most critical gestation period there is. Thank your body and trust that it knows exactly what to do to help you form this child. Although you may be transitioning out of fatigue and nausea, you may now start to get what is called "round ligament" pains. They do not last forever and happen toward the lower abdomen as you are stretching for your uterus to grow. Your belly may itch a bit during this period, and I found that lavender oil is both soothing and helpful. Your bump is expanding, so show it off! Your baby is creating a beautiful natural healthy glow around you that is obvious to everyone you meet, so enjoy the attention, and remember, you deserve it.

YOUR BABY ❧

A baby at thirteen weeks is fully formed and is starting to actually resemble a baby. The external genitalia have formed and so it is possible to tell if it's a boy or a girl! The eyes have moved closer together and your little sweetie has fingerprints now! Your baby is about three inches long, around the size of a potato, and can kick, bend, and suck his thumb.

YOUR SPIRIT ❧

Congratulations! You made it through your first trimester and you should feel elated. As your energy begins to weave its way back into your life, you will naturally feel lighter, happier and ready to take on the rest of your pregnancy. This is partly because people begin noticing you look pregnant, not so much because of your growing bump, but because of that super mama glow you have. This comes from within and emanates through you as you feel physically better and more emotionally ready to step into the next phase of your pregnancy. As you are starting plannig ahead for the next two trimesters, gathering your birth plan thoughts is an important part of cultivating your newly energized self. This planning needs time to mature and grow into exactly what you want it to be, so honor it by allowing enough time to get all details worked out. Start early and even if it does not go as planned, you will be comforted by these efforts and will have a foundation to work with no matter how your birth ends up.

WEEK 13 ⌒⌒

Pregnant women have an inner glow that shines through and radiates with positive energy and connectedness to the source of all beauty. When a woman carries life in her womb, she expands herself into the universal flow of energy, which awakens her senses and her inner spiritual energy. Growing a baby offers a woman the opportunity to be part of Mother Nature's mysteries, which directly connects her to the source of all things. When you live in balance with your body, mind, and spirit, your radiant glow is the external manifestation of this harmonious self-connectedness.

Reflections

This awareness may signal a time for you to reflect on what it means to be and look pregnant. Look at yourself deeply and take notice of how your energy flows and how you may see yourself differently. Remember that your growing baby brings a new life force to your body and your spirit, and this gift is an opportunity for you to look closely at how you manifest positive energy in your life.

Are you able to see your own "glowing" energy? Do you feel more spiritually connected now than you did before you were pregnant?

Bringing this positive balance to your life will only increase your ability to have an amazing pregnancy that will naturally lend itself to an easier birthing experience for you and your baby.

Ideas

· This topic may signal a great time to take some pregnancy photos that will document your journey through pregnancy. You may consider taking some pictures in nature where life energy is more abundant. This will help you to see how you and your baby are a part of the overall life force of the universe.

- Try exploring your deeper spiritual self by learning specific practices like meditation or yoga, or by reading up on various ideologies that have always held your interest.

Book Pairing

Joyful Birth: A Spiritual Path to Motherhood by Susan Piver

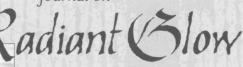Radiant Glow

Take time to journal about what
it is like to be pregnant and
how different your body is now
that you are growing your baby.
Write down how it feels to see
that "inner glowing" that only
shines through a healthy pregnant
mama, and journal about your
spiritual connection to this special time in your life.

hold your belly in gratitude

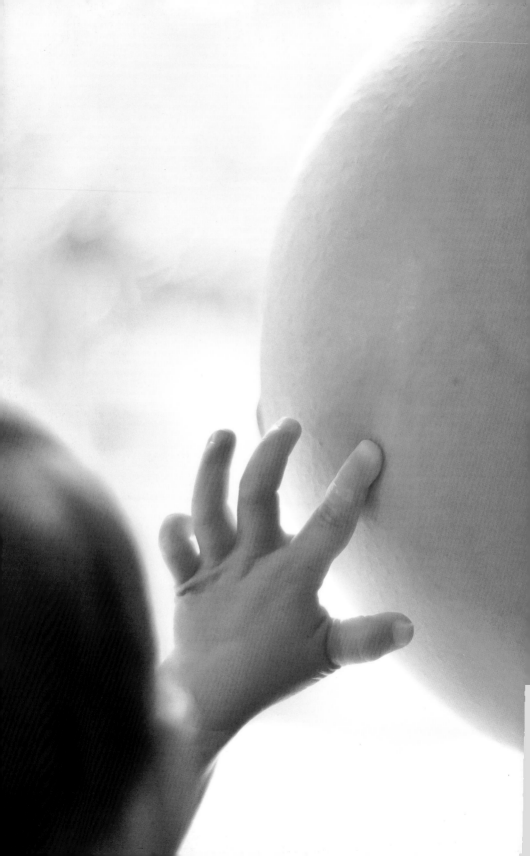

Bonding

*deeply connect with yourself
and your baby through spirit*

YOUR BODY ⚬〜

You are finally starting to feel more energized during this week and are definitely sporting a slight bump. As you finally begin "showing," it tends to make the experience more real and thus allows you the ability to really begin to bond with your baby. Take the time to literally feel your belly every morning, awakening your senses to this divine connection. *Remember to work at preventing uncomfortable symptoms rather than dealing with them.* So for example, drink a lot of water, around three quarts per day, and eat high-fiber and -protein foods to help with energy, stamina, and constipation. Fluids help prevent dehydration, headaches, and various infections that are common in pregnancy, so maintain this practice and make it a conscious part of your day. Try making up a pregnancy tea and keep it in the refrigerator labeled "mama tea only." Every time you open the fridge, have some. This "practice" ensures regular drinking throughout the day.

YOUR BABY ⚬〜

A baby at fourteen weeks is about the size of a small grapefruit, measuring in at around three and a half inches or so. All of the organs have developed and she is looking more and more human as the days pass. Your baby is obtaining all its sustenance from the placenta now and is basically hanging out and gaining weight, which also means weight gain for you. Welcome these changes and embrace all of the new energy and life your baby is breathing into your body.

YOUR SPIRIT ⚬〜

This week is all about connection—to your baby, to your higher self, and to your divine spirit. Bonding with your baby is only one aspect of this connection, as it is equally important for you to have a deep relationship with yourself. What does this mean? It means living in awareness so that your baby learns that what is important is how we care for ourselves and ultimately each other. Bonding and connection are not soundbites; they're part of a lifelong journey that grows and changes over the years. This week is a reminder to get to know yourself again and again, because as you change over the years, it's important to mark those changes so that you are open to the flow of your life. Becoming a mother is a redefinition. Even if this is your second or third child, each time you become a mother, you are redefined once again. In your daily meditations keep these connections alive and in your consciousness.

WEEK 14 ☙

What does it mean to be bonded to your baby? A mother and a baby have a connection like none other in the universe. You are the sole source that sustains your baby and your body is made to grow, birth, and feed a baby. This is the miracle of being a woman. Every mother in the universe knows that there is no other feeling like holding your baby for the first time. There are no words to describe that feeling and that deep connection that occurs. In that moment, time stops and everything in the world is perfect because you are holding *your* baby. Your instincts kick in and instantly you know what to do.

Reflections

Reflect on how you already feel about your baby. Are you connected or are you struggling with feeling bonded to your baby? Be honest with yourself. Even if you are not experiencing bonding feelings, it's important to take notice of this now, and not to judge yourself. Some women do not feel bonded to their babies before they are born—don't worry. You will love your baby just as much as every other mother does. You may need to hold your baby to feel that bonded connection. If you have other children, it's important to take time now to prepare your child(ren) for the new baby's arrival. Read books that talk about introducing a sibling to the family unit, consider allowing your child the responsibility of helping you name the new baby (or at least have input), and start to think about what your philosophy is on sleeping with the baby in a family bed and breast-feeding. These topics are important to think and talk about now so that when the baby arrives you have some idea how you want to approach these basic needs of your baby. Both breast-feeding and co-sleeping promote bonding with your baby, and it is important for you to determine your opinion on these issues.

Ideas

- Read up on co-sleeping with your baby and breast-feeding, and talk with your birthing practitioner about any concerns you have about these topics.
- Spend time every day talking with your belly and let your baby know he is loved. This practice is meaningful as you go down the road to actually holding your baby in your arms for real.

Kids' Book Pairing

Baby on the Way by Martha Sears, RN, and William Sears, MD
Welcome With Love by Jenni Overend

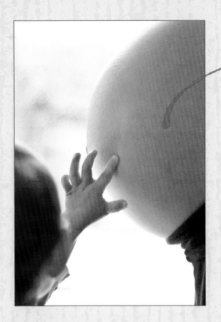

journal on

Bonding

Are you feeling bonded to your baby already? If not, do not be frustrated with yourself. Take the time to write about your feelings of connectedness to this baby.

deeply connect with yourself and your baby through spirit

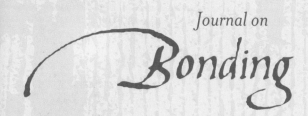

Journal on

Bonding

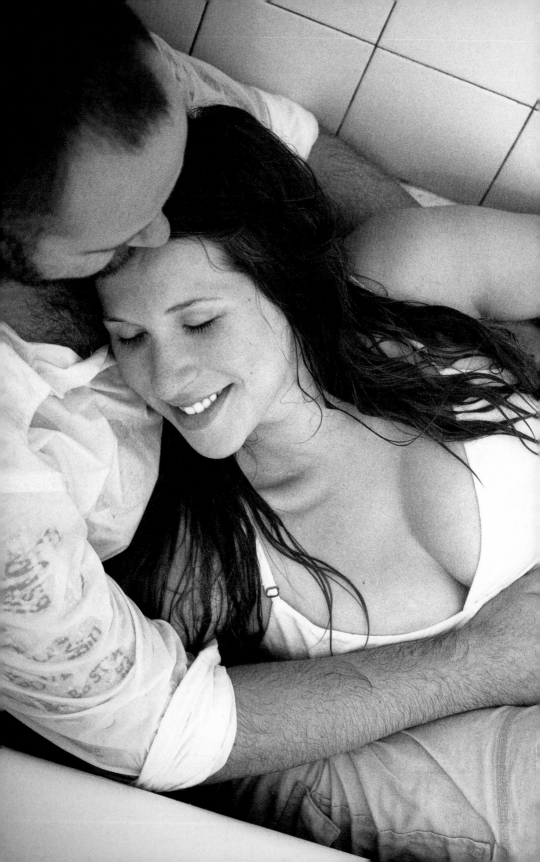

Partner Energy

honor the divine in all parents

YOUR BODY ❧

Many partners experience something called "sympathy symptoms" during the pregnancy and these are very real feelings both physically and emotionally and it's important to acknowledge these. He or she may have food cravings, gain weight, and even struggle with insomnia. Take time to talk with your partner about how he or she is feeling throughout the pregnancy seasons. The fifteenth week might signal some sleeping struggles and if that happens for you, try implementing a relaxing routine before bedtime, by doing a nighttime meditation, drinking a soothing pregnancy tea, or getting a light massage from your partner.

YOUR BABY ❧

Your baby at fifteen weeks is able to pick up sounds as his hearing is developing now, so both you and your partner should spend time talking to the baby and letting him get to know your voices. Keep your talking calm and loving so your baby feels little stress and is able to develop and grow in the loving tones of his parents. You may also begin to feel your baby move about now, but not feel really big kicks for a few more weeks.

YOUR SPIRIT ❧

Because you are feeling most of the physical symptoms of being pregnant, it can be hard to recognize that your partner is also feeling a number of things. Shifting the focus from you to your partner every so often takes some of the pressure off of both of you and allows for each of you to be heard and appreciated. This is a good practice, taking turns with needing "extra time" from the other, because after the baby comes, this will move from a nice way of being to an essential part of moving through those first days and weeks.

WEEK 15 ❦

You are carrying the baby and going through all of the physical symptoms, but your partner is also a HUGE part of this process and it's important to take time to acknowledge how he or she feels about the life changes involved with the arrival of the baby. Your partner may have anxious feelings about becoming a parent and be concerned about how to best support you in the birth. Include your partner in the monthly appointments with your midwife or doctor, and encourage him or her to ask questions. Remember that the two of you are in this together and each of you needs a space to vent, process, and learn.

Reflections

It is never too early to begin discussions with your partner about the many issues that having a baby can bring up. It's important for each partner to have a place to talk and process feelings when preparing to hold you and your baby in a space of strength as you birth the baby. Many partners do not know what to do to help the mothers through birth, but what is most helpful is communication. Say what you need and what you don't want. It's important to provide specific instructions so that your partner is prepared on the day of the birth and you feel supported in the ways that you need. Make sure that you talk about the kind of birth you are hoping for and that he or she feels confident to communicate those needs and desires to your birthing team if needed. Start asking questions about whether the two of you want others present at the birth, whether you want someone taking pictures or videos, or if you want it to be an intimate affair.

Ideas

- Ask your partner to write a letter to the baby expressing how she or he feels about her arrival.

- Encourage your partner to journal about becoming a parent and have a discussion about any fears around your birthing the baby.

- Ask your partner to write a list of all of your strengths as he or she sees them and keep that with you on your pregnancy altar and at the birth. You may turn that into a birth art project.

Music Pairing

"You Are The Best Thing" by Ray LaMontagne

Book Pairing

The Birth Partner by Penny Simkin and *Babyproofing Your Marriage* by Stacie Cockrell

journal on

Partner Energy

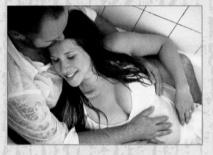

Take the time to write about how
this pregnancy is affecting your
partner and speak to the ways in
which you have included him or
her in this process. Allow your
partner to write in this section.

honor the divine in all parents

journal on

Partner Energy

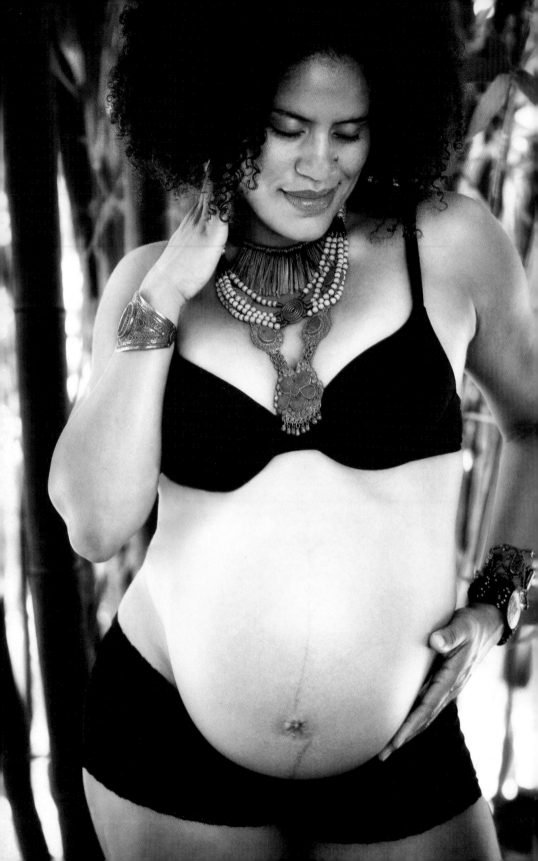

Sexy Mama

you are a sexy goddess—believe it!

YOUR BODY ❧

Let's start by just laying it out there: orgasms will not hurt your baby and they feel good to both partners. Your body needs stimulation, and sexual intimacy is one way this occurs during pregnancy. You have just made it through that first trimester of feeling tired and possibly sick to your stomach. So now that you are regaining some balance in your body, let loose in the bedroom. Let your body feel the pleasure of making love as you and your partner explore your newly shaped body and a deeper connection that exists because of your pregnancy. Your desire may come bouncing back threefold and if it does, just enjoy it! The only times you should worry about sexual intercourse are if you start bleeding or spotting, your water has broken, or if it's painful. In these instances, just consult your birthing practitioner for advice. Making love will also help with frequent leg cramps that may be plaguing you throughout the night.

YOUR BABY ❧

By sixteen weeks, your baby is about the size of a pear and her heart is pumping roughly twenty-five quarts of blood each day. Your baby now has eyelashes and is building super strong bones through the use of your calcium, so keep your calcium intake high. Your baby is well-protected in the cocoon of your placenta and will not be hurt by sexual intercourse. So do not let your baby stop you from enjoying yourselves.

YOUR SPIRIT ❧

So you made a baby, an intimate experience that started with two folks in love and ended with a new addition to your family. Now what? Are you spending time keep that flame burning now that you are pregnant or are you feeling sexually inhibited as a result of your growing belly and pregnancy ailments? Having sex with your partner during pregnancy is as important as maintaining the emotional intimacy between you. You do not have to worry about birth control.

WEEK 16 ⌇⌐

What do you see when you look at your body? Do you feel sexy and attractive? Do you feel like your partner likes your new curves and are you spending time connecting sexually? Being sexy means embracing your body as it changes and falling in love with your new, round belly. This new belly of yours is curvy and luscious because it contains the love you and your partner have for each other, your sweet little baby.

Reflections

You may be called to look deeply at your sexual history, especially before becoming a mother. Do you have sexually related issues that you need or want to work on? What is your relationship to sex, and have you ever had any sexual experiences that you feel need healing? These issues are important because working through them will allow for a meaningful sexual relationship with your partner and will help you to one day pass along healthy information on this topic to your own children. If you have experienced any sort of trauma in this area, you may want to consider talking to a psychologist about your experiences because birthing a baby can bring back a flood of memories that you may not want to recall. Working through any issues like this now is critical for a healthy birth experience for you and your baby.

Ideas

- Make love with your partner as much as you can, because it is true that after the baby comes, most of your time will be spent caring for the baby in those early days and weeks. This is a special time in your relationship, and taking the time now to really honor and worship each other will only make you a stronger family unit.

Book Pairing

Sexual Healing Book by Peter A. Levine

Music Pairing

"Beautiful" by Me'Shell Ndegeocello and "Sexual Healing" by Ben Harper

journal on

Sexy Mama

How is your growing belly affecting your sexual connection with
your partner?

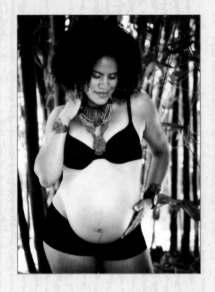

you are a sexy goddess—believe it!

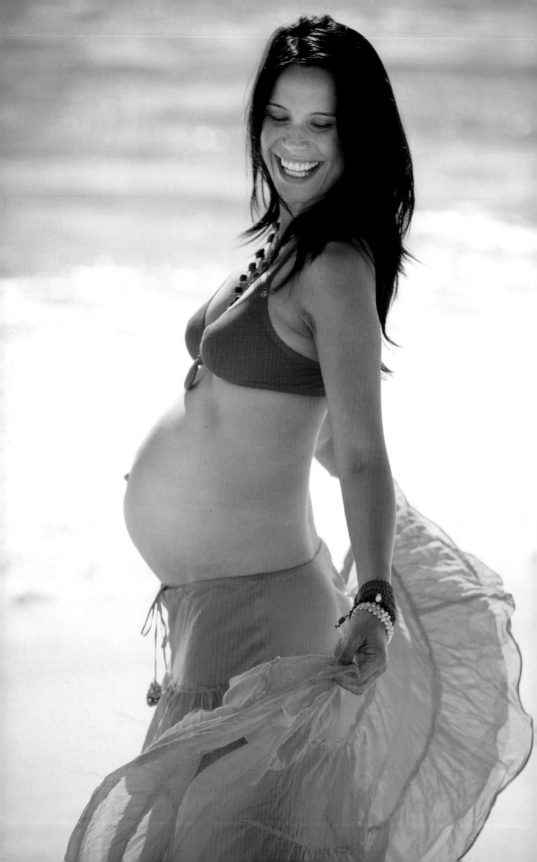

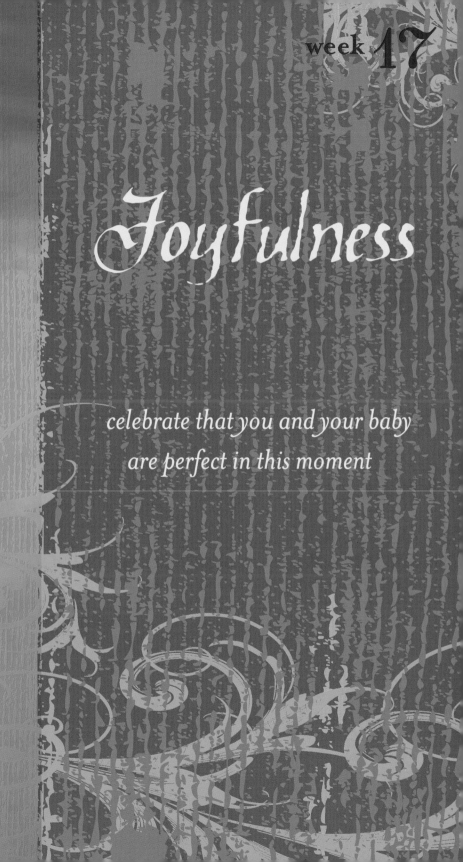

Joyfulness

*celebrate that you and your baby
are perfect in this moment*

YOUR BODY ❧

This week let's celebrate all that is happening in your body. This is a time to revel in the miracle of growing a baby and to set aside any uncomfortable symptoms so you can just enjoy this pregnancy. This week you should be feeling pretty good as long as you are drinking your fluids, eating well and sleeping at night. Your breasts are getting larger and preparing for the milk that will fill them to nourish and sustain your baby. I mean, can you believe that? Your body will provide the superfood your baby needs to live and grow into a healthy, little person. That alone is incredible.

YOUR BABY ❧

By seventeen weeks, baby is also happy to be growing inside of you. Your baby has chosen you, and that is something that only you can cherish. So do it! Your baby has reflexes, can swallow, blink, and suck. She is about five inches long and could fit nicely in the palm of your hand. Know that you have the perfect baby for you. In this moment, everything about you and your baby is perfect.

YOUR SPIRIT ❧

Have you ever stopped to think about why this particular little soul chose you and your partner for parents? What is it that you have to learn from one another? Take the time this week to marvel at all of the possibilities that await your new family. What are your hopes and dreams for your child and yourself as new parents? You are a parent now and remembering to cherish each moment of this very long journey with this little soul is just as important as every other part of this experience. Maybe even more important. The more joy you infuse into the process, the easier it will be.

WEEK 17 ❧

This is the week to celebrate! You are in what is typically considered the "easiest" part of the pregnancy, in that your energy has come bouncing back and your queasy period has passed. So feeling good and expressing gratitude should not be hard to do. Revel in your body's strength and ability to carry this baby, and really take the time to pay reverence to this gift.

Reflections

Women are born gifted! They can birth babies for heaven's sake. This is a magical and joyous event and something that, even though the medical community can tell us how it works, is incredible in so many ways. The fact that you can create a human life, carry it in your body, and birth it into existence is just so unbelievably miraculous that there are hardly words for it. Just take time to enjoy the fact that your body said yes! You have been gifted with a baby and it's time to scream it from the rooftops. Every single feeling of happiness and joy should be appreciated for this great happening in your life. So forget about all the pregnancy symptoms, and for this one week (and more if you can remember) just enjoy it all, even the aches and pains.

Ideas

- Write a letter to your baby letting her know how happy you are to become her mother.

- Write a letter to your own mother letting her know how you appreciate her bringing you into the world. This is just a happy and loving note, letting anything else just be set aside for this one simple act of appreciation. If your mother is deceased, honor her with a letter and take it to a place that reminds you of her and bury it in the earth.

- Live in gratitude for this baby. Perhaps do some birth art where you paint the words "I am grateful" and leave it on your pregnancy altar for a daily reminder of how much you appreciate the opportunity to become a mother.

Music Pairing

"I Give Thanks" by Katheryn Mostow

Any happy tunes by Ingrid Michaelson

journal on

Joyfulness

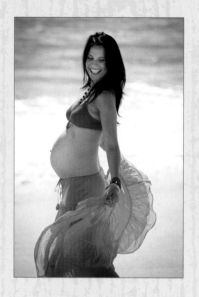

What are your favorite things about
being pregnant? Can you list them
and let your baby know the joy she is
bringing you?

celebrate that you and your baby are perfect in this moment

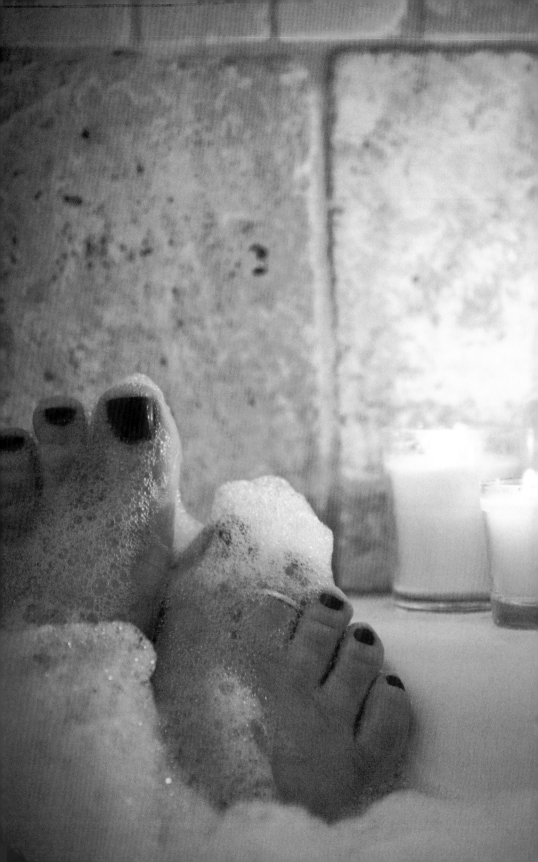

Nurturing Yourself

*indulge in pampering yourself
oh, c'mon, just do it!*

YOUR BODY ☙

This week is about indulging in a little extra nurturing for Mama's body and soul. I was always amazed when I would stand naked and look down and no longer see my feet. I knew in those moments that it was time for a little resting of my tootsies and a little soakin' of my bones. This is time to put on some great Bon Iver, Ray LaMontagne, or Patti Griffin, pour an extra helping of bubbles in the tub, and just soak. Read a book, besides this one, and just soak. Your baby belly might not be so big that you can't see your feet quite yet, or if it's your second or third baby you may have already hit that milestone, but nonetheless this week you deserve a little pamper-me time!

YOUR BABY ☙

By eighteen weeks, your baby is taking it a little easy on you, and just in time for the pamper-me fest. Your baby can hear you now, so make sure to let her know that mommy needs a relaxed week and that anything she can do to help you with that would be awesome. Your baby's bones are starting to harden and her senses are starting to develop so she will one day be able to experience all of the deliciousness life has to offer.

YOUR SPIRIT ☙

It's hard to keep going some days. When we take time to be nurtured and to nurture ourselves, it replenishes us. As mothers we give a lot of ourselves in every moment. We give of our body, our soul, our whole heart, and our knowledge. We have a big task when we agree with the universe to bring babies into the world, and being charged with such an awesome responsibility means we have to brave, courageous, kind, passionate, and protective every single day. That is a lot. So care for yourself, Mama. You deserve it.

WEEK 18 ☙

What does it mean to nurture yourself? Have you ever done it? Many women do not take the time to show themselves a little lovin' because they are too busy handing out the love cookies to others around them. Well if this sounds like you, it's your turn to dip your hand in that cookie jar and grab a bite. You may be the kind of person who does not allow your partner to do much for you, but try to allow him or her to do more. Remember that you are loved and maybe everything won't be exactly to your liking if you let your partner clean the bedroom, but let it happen anyway.

Reflections

Mama deserves a little pamper time, and let this be the week to indulge. Do you spend enough time giving to yourself or nurturing yourself? Most of us have super busy lives, so this does not happen very often. What stops you from just running down to your local spa and getting a massage? Carrying around a baby in your body is warrior work, and a little body lovin' can be just what you need to keep you going on this path. Most people can't afford it, but sometimes we have to do it anyway! Maybe this is the week you just say yes to yourself. We do not say yes enough to ourselves. Soon after the baby comes, everything will revolve around the baby's needs, as it should be, but you need to care for Mama too. Start practicing that now.

Ideas

- Take long bubble baths with sweet-smelling essential oils, such as lavender and grapefruit while burning your favorite candles. I love anything that smells like patchouli or brown sugar.
- Make homemade sugar scrubs for your face and feet. I make a chocolate face mask for my daughter and her friends that is also edible.
- If you can indulge in a professional pregnancy massage, do it! You deserve it.
- Stay in bed for a whole day just watching movies and eating with your partner, and throw in a little lovemaking session for good measure. A good orgasm goes a long way to relax and stimulate for your body.

Indulgence Pairing

Greenpad Living Soaps—yum!
www.greepadliving.com

journal on

Nurturing Yourself

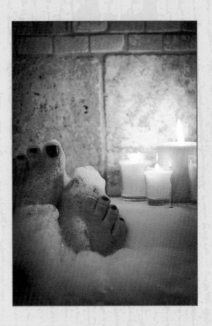

What are the ways in which you pamper yourself? What *really* makes you tick and feel good? Do you indulge in these things often? If not, why not?

indulge in pampering yourself
oh, c'mon, just do it!

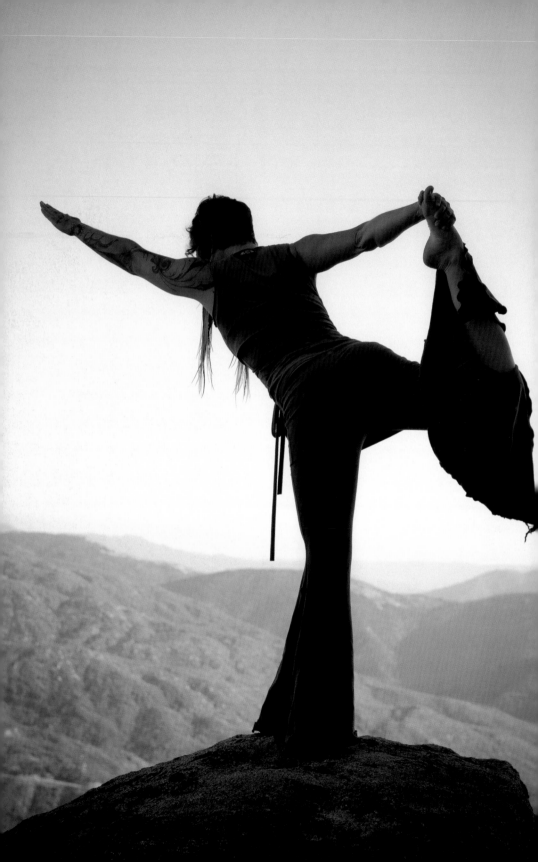

fear

love is stronger than fear

YOUR BODY ⌒

This week is about digging deep. Plain and simple, digging deep to find where you store the fears that keep you trapped in any sort of immobilization. Is it possible that you would not have any ailments if you lived in pure love without fear? These are merely questions worth pondering, but not judging. Notice in your body this week how it feels when you start to feel any fear around any issue related to his pregnancy. Do you feel differently than when you are completely relaxed and confident? Does it affect your mood swings? Panic is powerful, so don't nurture it. Feed your courage, feed your will, and feed your strength as a woman.

YOUR BABY ⌒

By nineteen weeks, the baby is about the size of a grapefruit and is developing vernix all over his body to keep his skin soft and protected from the amniotic fluid he is living in. Your baby can sense feelings and knows if you are happy, sad, or scared. Be in your courage place as much as possible so that when the big birthing day comes you two can work together and help him come into the world free of fearful energy and full of love and power.

YOUR SPIRIT ⌒

If you have never been pregnant before, you may be afraid of a whole bunch of things, but giving fear any energy is like feeding the savage beast. It gets hungrier, scarier, and more powerful. It's true that so many new and crazy things are happening to your body that it can be overwhelming. If you are indulging in a little light pregnancy book reading, you may have discovered every last detail of what could go wrong, but know this: whatever happens is your path and is meant to be. Trusting that the universe will only guide you down the path that is meant for you takes a lot of the stress and pressure off. Women have been birthing babies since the beginning of time and know how to do it, instinctually. Even if, by some stretch of the imagination, you did not have anyone at your birth except you and your baby, you would figure out what to do, because your body is made to do this work. Trust your inner knowing, do this emotional and spiritual work now of asking yourself all these hard questions so you can ready yourself to step into the ring with love as your sword and confidence your secret weapon. You can conquer all fear, with your will. You can do it.

WEEK 19 ⌒

Fear is the most powerful illusion there is.
—A COOL BUMPER STICKER I SAW ONCE

A beautiful singer I know named Aradhana Silvermoon wrote a song called "Love Is Stronger Than Fear," and it is so true. Within your deepest fear, you will find your deepest love too, and you can choose which will win in those moments. Love or fear? Our medical community has set birth up to be a big scary event that requires massive procedures, surgeries, and interventions. I have actually heard women say things like, "My doctor is going to *let* me birth naturally." Say what? Let you? Taking back our births as women is our right and our duty to our children.

Doctors are important in the field of birthing babies and they do save lives, but they have also fostered an environment of fear and disempowerment so that a woman will put all of her trust in the doctor without listening to herself. Inside and out, *you* know this stuff! Educate yourself, know what you are doing, and decide what tests you want to take and what ones you don't. Did you know you don't have to take any of the tests doctors offer if you don't want them and you don't ever have to be examined vaginally if you don't want that. I never had any tests done for either of the last two pregnancies and was never checked vaginally until my midwife showed up at my births.

Look at your own medical history, talk with midwives and doulas, do research, and take back your birth from the establishment. Even if you choose the hospital route, you have rights and you need to know them. It's your body, your baby, and your birth, and if you create a birth plan with your birthing team, your practitioner needs to follow that to the best of her ability, unless true complications arise. Women are being tricked into thinking that things like elective C-sections are okay. That is a major surgery girls and should never be the path *chosen.* Your baby has far less complications with breathing and nursing when she is born naturally through the vagina. A C-section was once for serious emergencies *only.*

Some women think if they have a C-section that they won't have to endure any birthing pain and that it will be easier, but that is the myth, sister! C-sections are far harder to recover from and are quite painful afterward. If you are a healthy mama, a natural drug-free birth can be yours for the low, low price of a few hours of focused energy, a little pain, and a lot of heart. You can do it, Mama! You can!

Reflections

What are your fears? List them all in a random stream of consciousness. It's important to get them out on a piece of paper so you can see them and determine whether any of them are based in reality. Are you afraid of giving birth? That it will hurt so much you won't be able to do it? Are you afraid that you will not be the mother you want to be? Where have you gotten your messages about pregnancy, birthing, and motherhood? Our culture doesn't support women in this process, but there are other women you can turn to for love and support. Check out *The Red Tent* movement if you are feeling alone or call places like Belly Sprout and talk to my friend Christy Funk. You can also call The Sanctuary Birth and Wellness Center (all listed under Resources on page 321). There is someone at each of those places who will be willing to hold your hand through this process. You are not alone. Join the Sacred Pregnancy community and one of the Sacred Pregnancy class series around the country. Women are gathering in circles to do this very important work—email me or join Ricki Lake and Abby Epstein's My Best Birth community. There is support out there. Just look up and you will see a hand waiting for you.

Ideas

- Research what works best for you and your family and writing your birth plan. A birth plan is just what your hopes are for the birth process. They should be flexible and open, but make your wishes known. Make sure to note whether or not you want any drugs and be specific about your goals for natural birthing. Also note how you wish to labor. This is especially important if you are in a hospital setting. Bring a birthing ball to the hospital for laboring, or let them know you wish to be in water (shower or bathtub) or that you want to walk around. Your birth plan belongs to you. Make it what you want and then be flexible when the day comes. Know your desires.

- Make a list of all your fears and burn them in a bonfire with lots of sage to mark the transformation of your fears into strengths.

- Make an "I can do it" sign to place on your pregnancy altar.

Music Pairing

"This Is Who I Am" and "Love Is Stronger Than Fear" by Aradhana Silvermoon

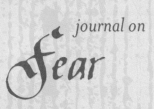

journal on
fear

After journaling your fears, write
how you can replace them with
power and strength. Use this space
to start jotting down notes for your
birth plan.

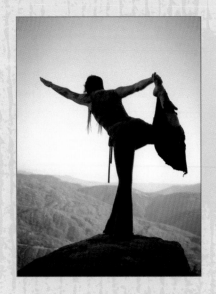

love is stronger than fear

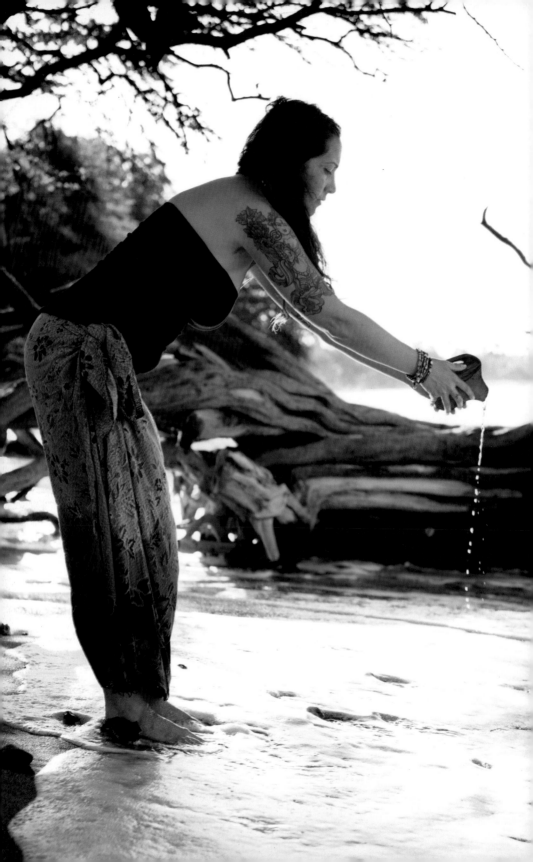

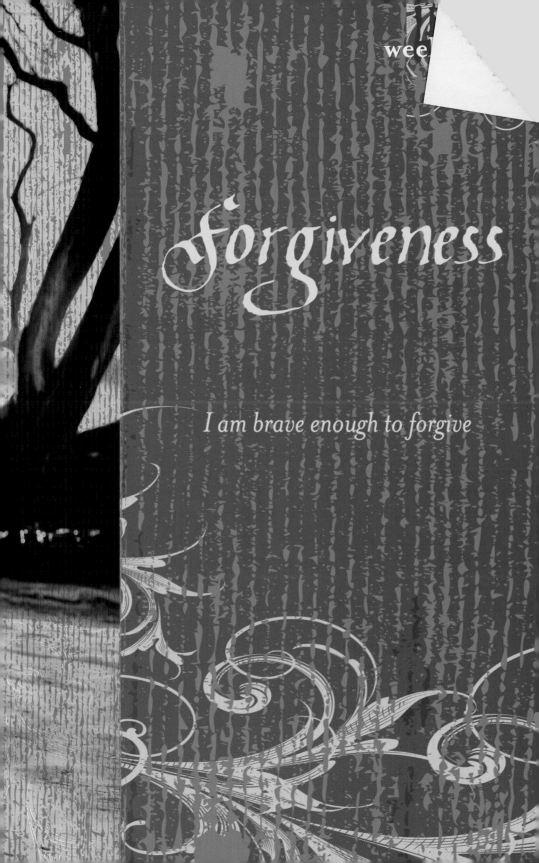

forgiveness

I am brave enough to forgive

YOUR BODY ❧

This is a big week because you are halfway there! At twenty weeks, your body is settled into the pregnancy and you are probably starting to feel little movements from your baby even though he is still less than one pound. You can decide around this time if you want to know your baby's gender or keep it a nice surprise until the end. What is great to focus on this week is healing any old wounds with the power of forgiveness so you are ready to invite your own child into your home in pure light and love.

YOUR BABY ❧

If you are getting an ultrasound during this twentieth week, and your baby is in the correct position, you should be able to tell if you are having a boy or a girl. I was told I was having a girl only to find out later that they were wrong, and I had a boy. So although the ultrasounds are pretty accurate, sometimes they are wrong or are read incorrectly. What is for sure is that your baby is counting on you to clear up any emotional junk so you can be present and awake for parenting him. All of the emotional work you do now will only help you create a more healthy relationship with your child in the future.

YOUR SPIRIT ❧

Being brave means so much more than being willing to endure whatever comes your way. In the book of true bravery, forgiveness is at the top of the list, because that is one of the hardest things to do and one of the most healing and powerful things to do. Becoming a parent means having to forgive yourself all the time because you're going to mess up—a lot! It's the nature of this journey, but being able to forgive yourself and your children when they mess up is a gift and a teaching. As a parent I strive to do better every day, but I make mistakes all the time. I try, however, to own them, to contemplate them so I can give an honest apology and then move on. We are all only human and by the nature of that fact alone, we are going to fall down. It's how we get up and the words we choose and the energy we put into the world that matters most. We teach our children life lessons of forgiveness by forgiving.

WEEK 20 ⌒⌣

This is the week to really look at your own childhood and see what you appreciated about it and what you might to do differently with your own child. For example, did you sleep in a crib or with your parents? Did you breast-feed or were you bottle-fed? Were you comforted as a baby or left to cry yourself to sleep? If you don't know the answers to these questions, find out. It's important to look into your own "babyhood" and determine how you want to relate and to care for your new baby.

Reflections

During this week of talking about forgiveness, what might you be holding onto from your past that you would do well to forgive and release? Did you have specific traumas as a child, like a parent leaving or a divorce, that left you unable to develop a relationship with the other parent that you feel has never truly been worked through? If you have experience big life transitions that you felt have gotten in your emotional way, now is the time to do some work on it. The more you can do now, the better you will feel going into motherhood.

Ideas

· Make a forgiveness tree! Draw a tree with branches and then cut out a bunch of leaves. On each leaf write something that needs forgiving in your life and attach it to the tree. Start each leaf with, "I forgive _____ for _____." This tree will represent the growth you have made throughout your life to get to the place where these things can be forgiven.

· Give the earth your tears! If you are really struggling with forgiving someone for doing something to you, a real trauma that is tough to just "let go" of, and you think this will hinder your parenting ability and you want to release it, take it to the earth. Mother Earth can contain your rage and tears. All you have to do is sit on the earth, ask for strength to forgive, find a rock to write your trauma on, throw it as far as you can from you, and ask for the earth to contain it so you don't have to. When you are done with this act and you walk away from it, *do not turn around and look back.* Move forward both physically and emotionally.

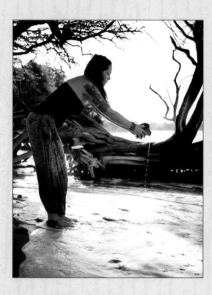

Forgiveness

Do you have childhood memories that need forgiveness? If so, what can you do to clear those cob-webs? Are you willing to release the past to start fresh with your own child?

I am brave enough to forgive

journal on

forgiveness

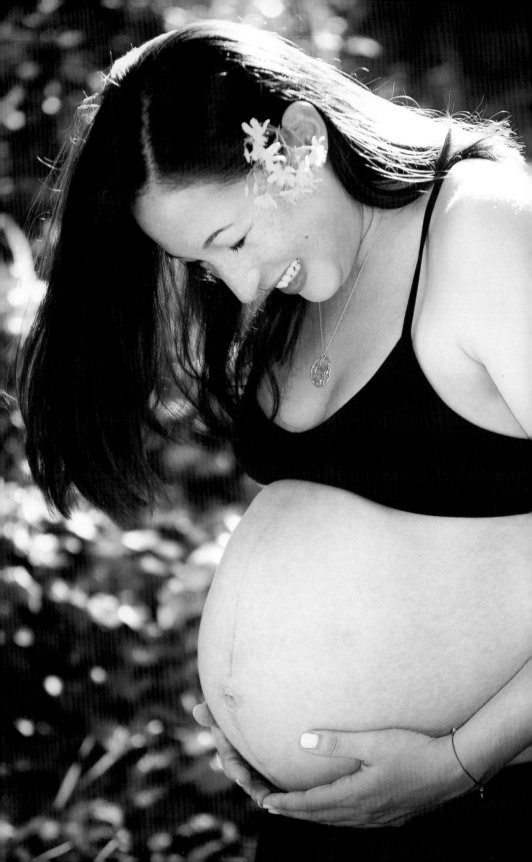

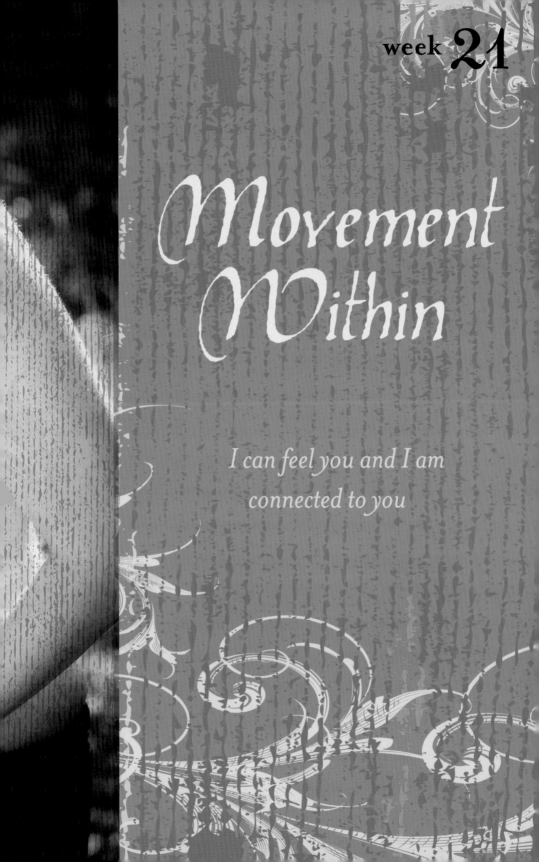

Movement Within

*I can feel you and I am
connected to you*

YOUR BODY ⌒

You are feeling a lot of symptoms this week and may even start seeing a few stretch marks coming your way. Not every woman gets them, but if you do, try massaging your belly with Vitamin E oil and increase your intake of Vitamin C. Stretch marks happen because your skin is stretching to accommodate the baby and they are typically hereditary. So if your mom got them, there is a good chance you will too. You may notice that you are now extremely hungry all the time. Your baby needs food and sustenance to grow and be healthy, and so do you. Eat foods that are rich in protein so you can feel more full for longer periods of time if the constant snacking is getting on your nerves.

YOUR BABY ⌒

Your baby is having a bunch of fun in there, moving, playing, and getting taste tests of all the food you eat. This is why it's very important to concern yourself with your choices. Your baby is actually using her taste buds to learn about flavors, so help her shape up his palate now. She is about the size of a pear now and is very interested in all that you are doing.

YOUR SPIRIT ⌒

When asked their favorite thing about being pregnant, many women have said feeling the baby move. There is something so magical about that feeling. It excites you, brings you joy, and helps you feel more connected to the baby. It can be difficult to know how to relate to your baby, when you cannot see her or hold her, but her movements are her way of talking to you and letting you know she is there and excited to be growing inside you.

WEEK 21 ⌒

Listening to your baby's movements can also tell you a lot about her. My third baby Bodhi was a constant mover in my belly, at night and during the day! It seemed like he never stopped moving around. I started to talk with him, asking him to calm down at night so I could rest. He accommodated me sometimes, but most often not. It turns out Bodhi is the one child of mine who is extremely active. From the moment he opens his eyes in the morning to when he shuts them at night, he is going! He loves to run, kick balls, dig, climb, and generally anything that keeps him moving. So if you pay attention now, you may get a little glimpse into what you child will be like later.

Reflections

How does it make you feel to actually know that you are carrying a baby in your body and what are your thoughts when you feel her move? Toward the end of your pregnancy, your baby gets pretty cramped inside of you, so when she moves, it's fun to see a little foot kick out your belly or an elbow on your side or see your entire belly moving around, as your baby turns and shifts to get comfortable. This is fun to include your other children in to get connected to the baby as well. As soon as you feel a kick, invite small hands to cover your belly to see if they might also get a little hello from baby. Make sure to tell your children to talk to the baby and introduce themselves to her, so she will know who they are when she arrives. It is super exciting to see your other children light up when "their baby" kicked them from inside mommy's tummy.

Ideas

- Play games. Tap on your belly lightly on one side and then the other side to see if your baby responds with kicks and movement. You can also do this with a flashlight that is on from side to side to see if they respond to light.
- Journal about when you first felt your baby move. This could be fun information for your child to have later on.
- Cool Fact: The woman in the picture on page 154 actually felt her baby girl move at the exact moment when Alexandra took that shot. Amazing!

journal on

Movement Within

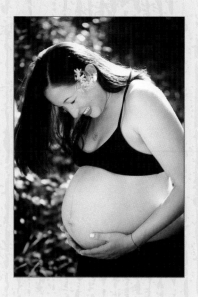

What was it like to feel your baby
move for the first time? Did it
make you feel more connected to
the baby?

I can feel you and I am connected to you

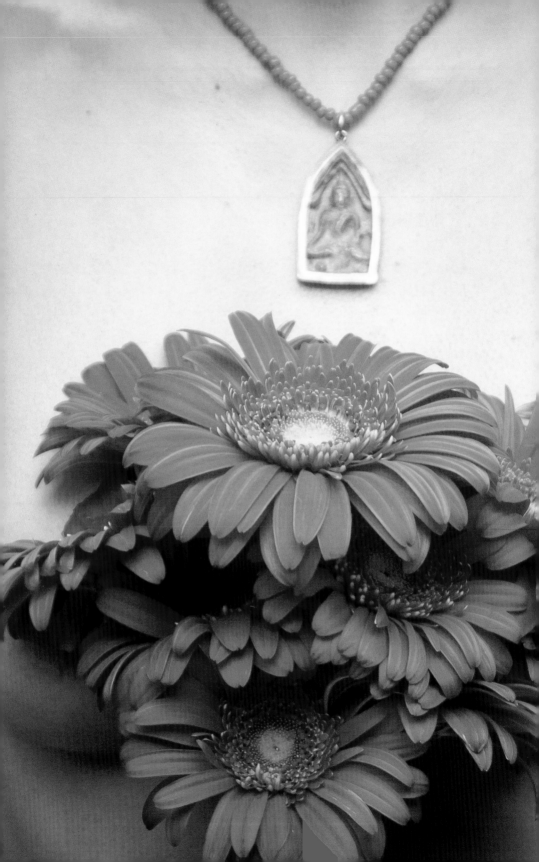

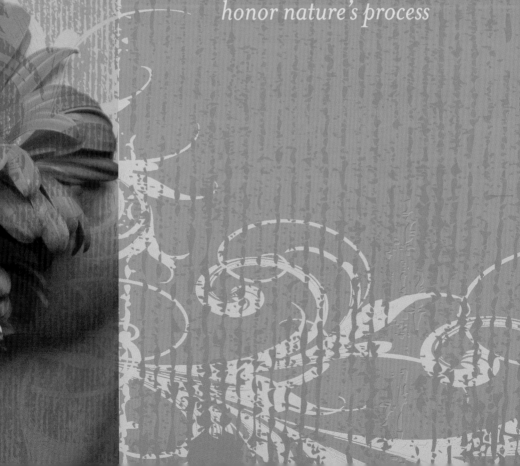

trust

honor nature's process

YOUR BODY ❧

Your belly bump is growing bigger, you "look" pregnant and are probably feeling emotionally better as your hormone levels are balancing out now. Your cravings may be subsiding and you are just steadily eating and gaining weight for your little one to grow. Try to remember to keep your feet up every night for a little while. This is important as you embrace your new body with a trusting willingness to gain as much weight as your baby needs, and always remember that your body knows exactly what it needs to create your baby as you work in perfect sync with each other.

YOUR BABY ❧

A baby at twenty-one weeks is moving all around in the amniotic fluid now and is probably kicking you like crazy. He is about the length of a banana and can respond to sounds and will really start to get used to hearing all of the voices around him. Talk to your baby a lot more now and encourage your partner and his siblings to do the same. Your baby will be born knowing everyone in his family simply by hearing your voices now.

YOUR SPIRIT ❧

Inhale trust ... exhale fear! Inhale trust ... exhale fear! Once more, inhale trust ... exhale fear! You are essentially at the midpoint of your pregnancy and because your morning sickness has passed a while ago, you have more time to focus on preparations for yourself, the birth, and the baby. Growing a baby requires so much trust and release from fear. When you let nature work how she is supposed to, things always work out beautifully. Birthing has become a fear-based institution, stripping women of their internal knowledge that their body knows how to perfectly create a baby. This has been replaced with test after test and books that are filled with advice that goes directly against mothering instincts. What are your fears? Sit with them, make friends with them, and then politely ask them to leave. Bringing this level of release to your awareness now will set you up for a lovely transition into motherhood.

WEEK 22 ⊙⌢

Trust is a big concept and something that most people struggle with. Trust is so hard to put into practice. When we blindly trust, we cannot know what the outcome will be. We have no control, and that is very scary for many people. When a woman gets pregnant, her baby begins to grow and is 100 percent trusting. The baby can only communicate with you through movement and is simply relying on you to do all of the right things and to step into motherhood, pure and confident. This is a monumental lesson in trust. All you can do is believe that your baby will grow into a happy, healthy being. You cannot force it to happen, only trust. If you have fears about going through the birthing process, have faith that this is an ancient rite of passage that many women have gone through before and you will too. Your body knows what to do and your strength will shine through as you deliver your baby into the world.

Reflections

It is time for you to look deeply within to see how you believe in yourself and the mysteries of the universe.

Meditate on how you deal with trust vs. fear and which normally wins that argument in your head. During your pregnancy, you are called upon to have confidence that your baby is growing perfectly and that you will be able to deliver your child with ease and in harmony with the universe. Remember to believe in yourself and the universal plan that all things happen for a reason. As life lessons can be learned with each experience, every act is a gift.

Ideas

· Think about the times that you have really trusted yourself, and times when you have not. What was the difference?

· Practice trusting! Start with small things, like believing that the foods you eat are helping to form your healthy, strong baby and work your way up to truly believing that your birth experience will be painless and your baby will enter the world in the arms of peace and love.

- Create a trust wheel: draw a circle and write who and what is allowed in. You may then say or write that anyone or anything else needs your permission to enter into your sacred space.

Website Pairing

Trust Birth
www.trustbirth.com

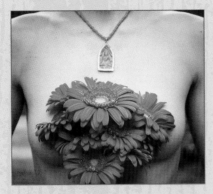

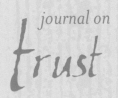
Take time to write about what
you are having trouble trusting in
regard to your pregnancy. Are
you concerned that you will not be able to let go during birth and
have faith in yourself to birth your baby? Journal these thoughts and
remember to believe your intuition!

honor nature's process

journal on

trust

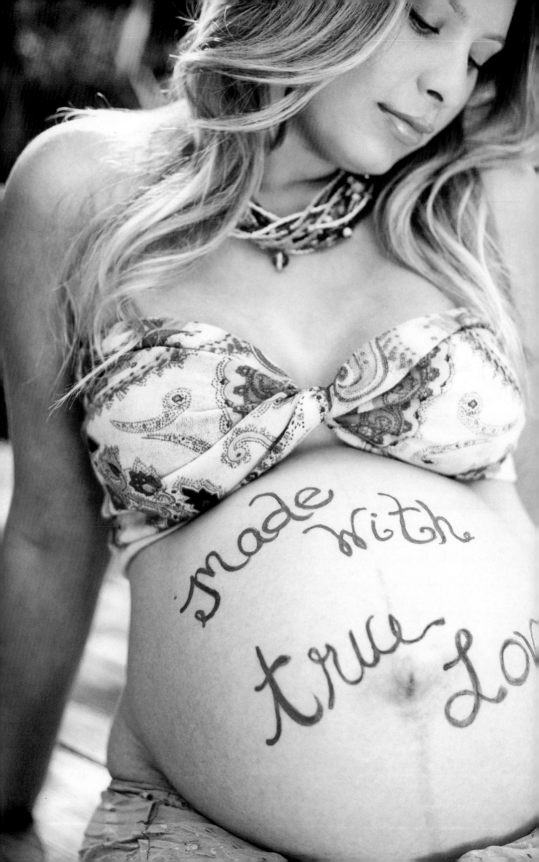

Baby Girl

my daughter will one day be
a powerful woman

YOUR BODY ❦

This week focus on loving your body and the fact that you are woman and *can* have a baby. There are many women who cannot carry a baby for various reasons. Take a moment to put aside ailments to live in gratitude for your awesome body's ability to take on this task. If you are feeling particularly moody or emotional this week, try to bring this gratitude to the forefront of your thoughts. You will be gaining weight like crazy and possibly struggling with sleep. At night, allow your mind to drift off in meditation about becoming a mother to a little baby girl.

YOUR BABY ❦

Your baby at twenty-three weeks is ready to give you a mini-preview of what is to come. You may start feeling those Braxton Hicks contractions more and more, but don't worry about them. This is a normal part of your pregnancy working hand in hand with the universe to prepare you to meet your baby. Your little girl is about eight inches long and still super pink.

YOUR Spirit ❦

This week spend time contemplating your life with a little girl. You're having a daughter, someone to bring into the sisterhood embrace and someone who will quite possibly one day carry a baby of her own in her womb. Make a vow, right here and now, that she will not be plagued by societal "girl" standards and that Barbie will not be her ideal. Vow that she will love and cherish her body because you will teach her that she is beautiful no matter what and that all those models on all those magazines are beautiful, yes, but imperfect. Help her to see the wisdom in knowing who she is and following her heart. This is an awesome task, but you can do it. She picked you to carry her through the trials and tribulations of "girlhood," so be humbled and say, "YES!"

WEEK 23 ⌒

Have you wondered what kind of mother you will be to a little girl vs. a little boy? Will there be any differences? What are your hopes and dreams for your daughter and how might you help her unfold into the person she is meant to be? Spend some time this week giving some thought to your sleeping arrangements. As you talk through these issues with your partner, what are you hoping to do with your baby after she is born? Will you hold her in your arms all night long or lay her in a crib? What feels right to you as a mother? I remember falling asleep that first night with my first son lying in my arms in our bed and waking up to see his gorgeous face and just loving every moment of snuggling and breast-feeding him. From that moment on, I knew we had wasted our money on the crib we had bought him. He never slept in that crib and since then none of my children have ever used one. We have what has warmly been termed "a family bed." Some nights it's all of us but my teen in the bed, and sometimes he even comes on in to join the fun. Although there are nights I crave a little alone sleeping time, I would not trade sleeping with my kids for anything in the world. Those are moments that I will forever cherish. All the feet in the face and the elbows to the back are worth it. Kids are little for only a minute really and adults forever. Cherish the time while you have it!

Reflections

When I was pregnant with my second child, we went in for my one doctor appointment toward the end of my pregnancy for an ultrasound. Having a home birth, you see a midwife every month and usually have one appointment at the end with a doctor. He did the ultrasound and then asked me if we wanted to know the gender of the baby. My little six-year- old son was there at the appointment and he *really* wanted to know, so we told the doctor it was okay to whisper it to my son. Ten seconds after *he* got the news, he blurted out, "We're having a sister!" We were all overjoyed. I realized at that moment how much I wanted a girl. Of course we said the same thing everyone says, "As long as we have a healthy baby, it doesn't matter," and to some degree that was true. However, in all honesty, I wanted a daughter and in that moment I realized how much. I went on to have two more sons after my precious daughter was born and am grateful for each one of my kids, but I am happy that I have a chance to mother a daughter and that I have someone to pass down my womanly knowledge to. I like that I can keep that circle going and that the power of woman lives in this household of boys.

What are your thoughts on having a girl? Do you have a preference and if you do, does that make you a bad person or ungrateful? This is all just information to process and think on. If you already know that you are indeed having a daughter, how do you feel about it? What is your relationship to other women like? What messages about being a girl did you get growing up? Were you taught to be strong and full of fire and to love being a girl or not given any girl wisdom to help guide your path? How will you help her cross over her life stages and rites of passage? Will you mark those and help her know what honoring girl-hood is all about?

Ideas

- Write a poem to your daughter. In it, pass along your woman wisdom to her and tell her how she is entering a very sacred tribe of sisters and to be proud of being a girl.

- Make her a necklace that you will give to her one special, random day. Then on that day, you can tell her about the pregnancy and birth and how honored you are to have had a daughter.

- Research sleeping options for your baby and you. Pick what feels right to you or just wait until she arrives and see what fits for your family. Listen to your instincts and know that as a mother you will know what is the best thing to do.

- What will the first words to your baby be? Write them down so you won't forget what you wanted to say upon meeting her.

Music Pairing

"Soul Sister" by Cree Summer
"Daughters" by John Mayer

Book Pairing

Raising Girls by Steve Biddulph

journal on

Baby Girl

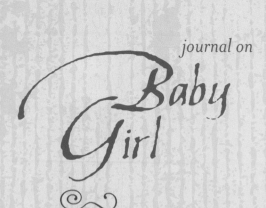

How do you feel about the potential of having a daughter? What is your relationship to other women like? How do you see yourself parenting a little girl?

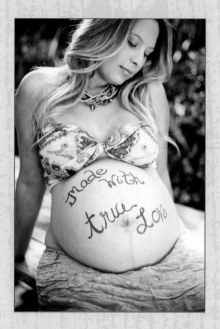

my daughter will one day be a powerful woman

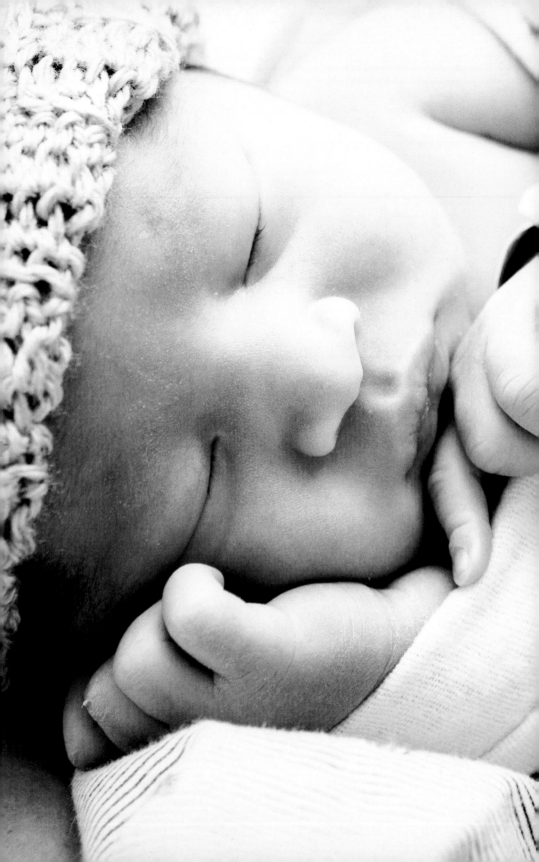

Baby Boy

my son will be kind, caring,
and full of life

YOUR BODY ⌒

This week, bring your focus to life with a baby boy. What does that
mean for you and your family? Boys tend to be bigger at birth, so
you may be hungrier and need to allow yourself a few extra pounds,
which means a bigger belly, which means a lot of touches. How do
you feel about strangers approaching you and touching your belly? I
believe that people who see a big, beautiful, round, pregnant belly just
instinctively reach out to be a small part of the magic and mystery of
pregnancy and birth, and I do not think they are any less than well-
meaning. Try to take unsolicited touches with a grain of salt and perhaps be grateful that so many are reaching out to bless you and your
baby's journey.

YOUR BABY ⌒

Your baby at twenty-four weeks is weighing in just over one pound
and is starting to be able to deposit fat into his body, so he will get all
plumped up before coming out to meet you. At twenty-four weeks,
if your baby was born prematurely, he could have a shot at surviving.
Your baby boy is also able to suck this hand or thumb on purpose if he
chooses to and has his lungs nearly developed.

YOUR SPIRIT ⌒

This week, spend time contemplating your life with a little boy. What
does it mean to have a son? You are blessed with the responsibility of
raising this boy into a good man. A man who cares deeply about others and who might one day be a father. You have so many adventures
in store for you with a little boy and a lot of mud, dirt, climbing, and
running. Mostly, though, you have a gentle soul who will cherish you
as his mother and whom you will need to offer your whole heart. How
does your partner feel about having a son? Keep the lines of communication open as you go through these last weeks.

WEEK 24 ⵏ

What are your hopes and dreams for your son and how might you help him to unfold into the person *he* is meant to be? Spend some time this week giving some thought to whether or not you will circumcise this little boy. To date, there is no real medical reason to do it and many folks think this is an archaic ritual that has no place in modern society. It is extremely painful for your son, and really consider if it's worth it to you to have this procedure done. Make sure, if you do not want it done and you are having a hospital birth, that you make your wishes known in your birth plan.

Reflections

I have three sons and can tell you first-hand that each one, while raised in the same house with the same parents, are very different. Each is unique and special and brings something else to our family table. I love that boy energy that permeates our home and know that these boys will do good in the world and will live by their hearts. It's a hard path to navigate. There are so many unique things about boys, so if you are having one, read up and decide how you think they need to be parented.

What are your thoughts on having a boy? What is your relationship like with your own father? Do you have brothers and are you used to all of the very "boy" things that are likely to come with this little bundle? How do you feel about a muddy, messy house? It's a good idea to think beyond babyhood because it lasts for about a minute, and then comes toddler land and beyond—boys like to bring in the dirt! (Girls do too, but you might see just a tad more muddy trails hanging off the boots of your sons.) If you are the type of person who *has* to have a clean home, you may want to work on that issue now. The more you can release around having a super sparkling clean home, the better. It's a lot of pressure on you and the child to maintain that level of perfection. Childhood, like life, is a messy event and it really should be. When my boys come home from school muddy from head to toe, I know they had a great day and that is the best thing I can ask for.

Ideas

- Write a poem to your son. In it, pass along your hopes and dreams for him.
- Make him a necklace that you will give to him just one special random day. Then on that day, you can tell him about the pregnancy and birth and how honored you are to have had a son.
- Research circumcision this week. Get all the facts before you decide what you want to do on this issue.

Music Pairing

"Sitting on the Dock of the Bay" by Otis Redding

Book Pairing

Raising Boys by Steve Biddulph

I Love Dirt by Jennifer Ward

Baby Boy

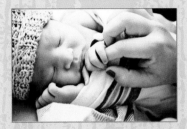

How do you feel about the potential of having a son? What is your relationship to men like? How do you see yourself parenting a little boy?

my son will be kind, caring, and full of life

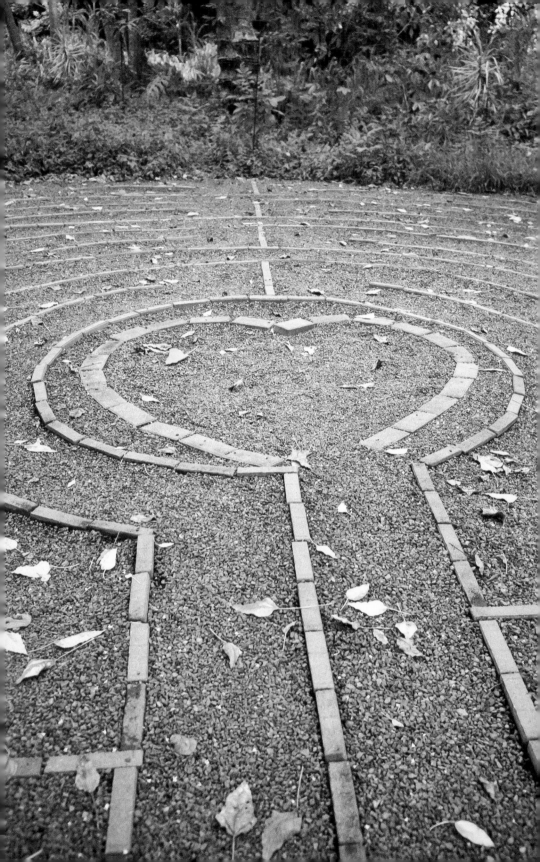

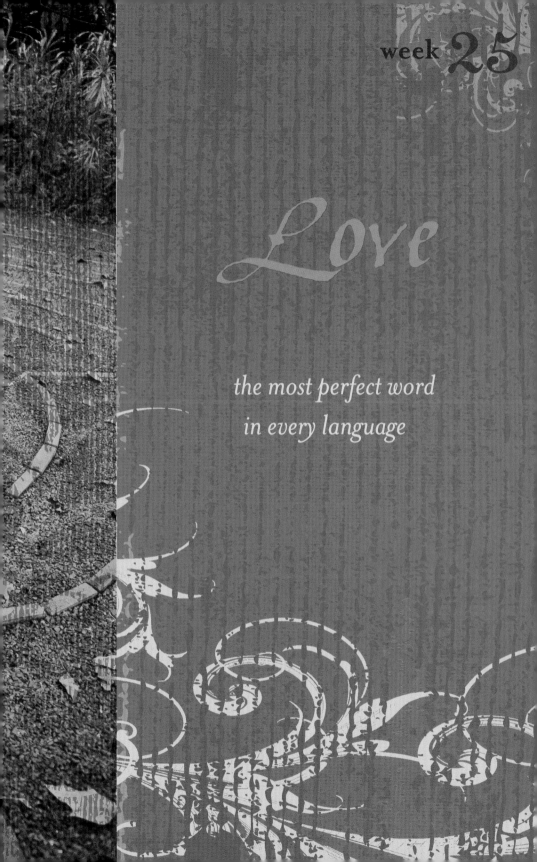

Love

*the most perfect word
in every language*

YOUR BODY ❧

Your body works hard for you and your baby—show it some love this week! Kick your feet up every day, even if it's only for a few moments. If you can get one of those yummy pregnancy massages, do it! Your back is likely to be feeling sore as your front weight is heavier now and it places pressure on your back. Practice good posture, do those Kegel exercises and get lots of warm, soothing baths.

YOUR BABY ❧

You are almost done with your second trimester and the good news is if your baby happened to be born prematurely at twenty-five weeks, the rate of survival is good. Your baby is pretty developed by now and is really spending these last weeks gaining weight and filling out those lungs and that body fat.

YOUR SPIRIT ❧

Do you remember falling in love with your partner? The amazing euphoria new love brings? Well brace yourself—because if you think that was cool, wait until you hold your little darling for the first time. Love is the most healing feeling in the world—it can literally cause wars or bring nations together. That is serious stuff. The power of your love is what will grow your child's essence, her soul, and only you and your partner can provide that kind of lovin'. Sure, many others will join in this love fest of your little baby, but it will be different than what you provide. Your baby will not thrive without your love, touch, and all those oogles over her. She needs to be the center of your universe so she knows the world is a safe and loving place that she can feel good about joining. I was reading a book somewhere that said that you don't want to spoil your baby with too much affection, and I about died. I could not believe those words were out in the universe being offered as "good advice." I don't know it all, but sister, this I do know. You can *never* give your baby too much love, too much attention or too many kisses and cuddles. You may try, but you won't be able to. They are the most delicious beings in the world with their pure energy, and I cannot imagine a world where I stopped loving on my kiddos.

WEEK 25 ⌒

Love is life and is what makes the world go round. Love is the one universal language that everyone around the whole world can speak and the love for a child is a singular feeling that cannot be compared to anything else. My kids and I play this game where I will say, "I love you more than all the chocolate in the whole world" and then Bodhi will say, "I love you more than all the shells on the beach in the whole world" and we go back and forth playing the "I love you more than … " game. I think having children makes your heart, or your ability to love, grow, because the love a mother has for her child is something that exceeds all other connections. It's the kind of love that creates energy in the exhausted momma so that she can hold her sick baby throughout the night, the kind of love that builds strength as you have to carry around an infant, all kinds of gear, and snacks. It's the kind of love that knows no bounds as your screaming toddler yells and screams he won't do what you are asking and you just scoop him up and wrap him in your love to see what is *really* going on with him. Motherhood is not for the faint-hearted oh no, it's for the brave and fearless. When you love like this, you can have your heart broken again and again, but the journey with these little ones is so worth it!

Reflections

After I had my first child, I worried that I would not be able to love subsequent children as much as my first—I mean, how would that even be possible? Then I had my daughter and my love affair with her just started all over again. It happened. I *did* love her just as much— and then the same thing occurred with my two other sons. Each child brings something new to your family den and honestly it's not something you will know until it just happens. This concept is a feeling and therefore tough to describe, which is why people have used poetry and attempted to string together the most beautifully dripping words to *try* to explain it. In reality, however, it's a feeling and not a thought, so try not to overthink this one. If you are afraid, as some women are, that you might not love your baby after she is born, release that fear. You will. Do not judge yourself for exploring all of your thoughts, but know that this baby-love thing is just out of your hands. You will love your little sweetie no matter what and you will become a lioness of protection. Your kisses and snuggles will save the world. Breathe into the love that you will feel for her and she will feel for you. This is also a reminder to love yourself! You are doing an amazing feat, Mama, take time to really fall in love with you too!

A LETTER TO MYSELF *by Connie Hozvicka*
FROM DIRTY FOOTPRINTS STUDIO

Dear Connie,

Let's be honest.

Lately you've been feeling super crappy.

I know. You're in a constant state of nausea, your mind is a tad bit foggy, you break into hot flashes at yoga, and saying that you're always exhausted is a bit of an understatement. And I know, this is really hard for you—because you're not feeling yourself and you're getting so far behind on everything. Emails, blogging, workshops, keeping everything in order. I know, I know, I know—you're always so good at doing what you do—but now, you feel like you're slipping. You feel like you're losing ground. And yes, I know you're worried. You're worried that all that you've worked so hard on with Dirty Footprints Studio is going to fall apart.

Don't be silly, Connie. Okay? Just stop it.

Worrying takes you out of total alignment with Creative Source, and it's not good for the baby.

And listen, your readers will understand. Most of them are mothers themselves—mothers that you've always admired and wondered how the hell do they do it all.

And you know what, Connie—you're gonna be fine. You're gonna be better than fine. You're gonna thrive—and have so much fun—and feel more blessed than you ever have in your whole entire creative, juicy life.

But now, you just need to take care of you. Listen to your body. Surrender to your body. It knows what to do—so let it. Rest when it asks you to—eat when it says you're hungry—

and keep sipping that delicious peppermint tea. You'll be through this first trimester stuff in a jiffy—and have more energy again. Promise.

And until then, let me take care of things. Okay? That's what I'm here for in the first place.

BIG hugs,
your higher self

Ideas

- Write a love letter to yourself this week! Encourage yourself to work through any places where you feel stuck this week!

Book Pairing

Guess How Much I Love You by Sam McBratney

Movie Pairing

Babies documentary and *Shakespeare in Love*

journal on

Love

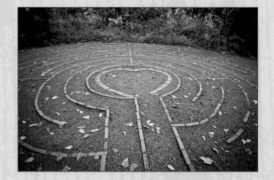

Use this space to write
that love letter to yourself!

the most perfect word in every language

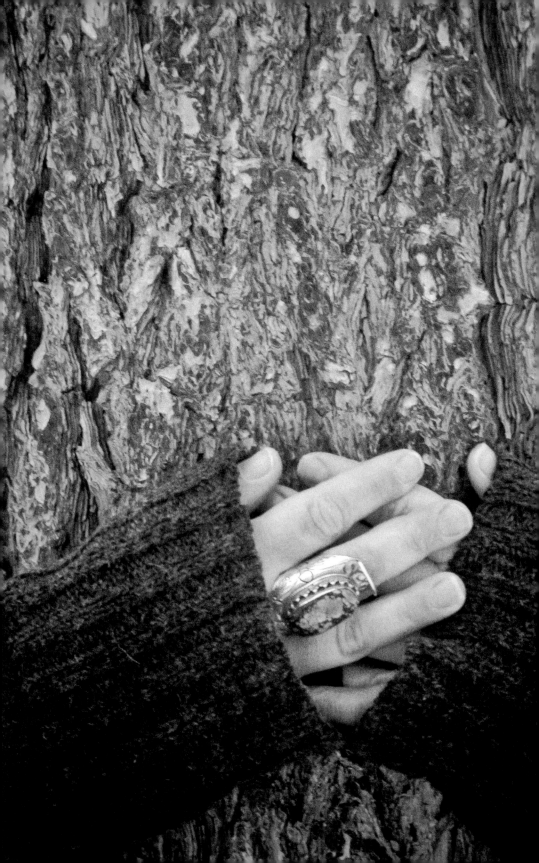

Earth Energy

we are all connected

YOUR BODY ❧

You may be having trouble remembering stuff and although this is a normal part of pregnancy and temporary, it might be frustrating to you as you go through the days. Ask Mother Earth for her help in giving you more balance as you navigate these last weeks if you feel increasingly off-kilter. Stand firmly on the earth as much as humanly possible and soak up the energy and power of Mama Earth.

YOUR BABY ❧

Your baby at twenty-six weeks is a big kicker and you may even have trouble sleeping as a result of these movements. There is still plenty of room in your uterus for baby to move around, so she will move and shake as much as possible. Try adjusting your sleep position slowly in order to make yourself more comfortable. Your baby is around two pounds now and is beginning to see and blink. Your new little one is the ultimate gift from the universe and it's important to see how your baby will fit into the earth's plan and your new family life.

YOUR SPIRIT ❧

If you have not already signed up for birthing classes, now may be the time to check it out. Check the Sacred Pregnancy website to see if there are any Sacred Pregnancy birthing classes happening in your area. If there are not, you may also try hypbirth, Lamaze, or Bradley classes to help you prepare to ground and find the inner strength to carry you through these last weeks and ultimately through the birth. Ask your birthing team to help you find a class if you are struggling finding one.

WEEK 26 ❧

The element of Earth reminds you to be grounded and centered during your pregnancy. When you have a reverence for Mother Earth, she allows you to borrow resources from her in your time of need. If you do not live in a natural environment, take a day trip to nature where you can really spend time feeling the earth with your toes and bow-ing to the ultimate mother creator. When you see how massive nature is and how she cares for her earthly children, you realize you are a part of the fabric that makes up the collective. You are just as strong as a 100-year-old oak. If you feel weak, ask Mother Earth to be there by your side and she will. Ask the old oak tree to be there to hold you up when you feel like you are falling down, and she will. Ask the sturdy rocks who contain all earthy memories to give you the gift of steadfast calm when you are charged with birthing your baby.

Reflections

You are one person among millions, and you are here because the earth supports you. We are taught about caring for our little ones by our Mother Creator, who cares so well for us. Show her some respect this week. Give up a day of your "regular" life to help clean her up, pick up trash on a beach, water the garden, take pictures of fields of flowers, give back in some small way in honor of the huge gifts you get every day. We want a healthy planet for our babies to grow and crawl and run on, and we must do our part to keep her clean and happy. Mother Earth is the ultimate supporter of us all, and she will be there for you when you are ready to birth your baby.

Ideas

- Spend time with Mother Earth, in nature, touching the trees, collecting fallen leaves, and letting your feet be bare upon her back.
- Find a rock that you can take home from one of your favorite nature spots, decorate it, keep it on your pregnancy altar, and bring it to the birth. Collect leaves and glue them into this journal.

Website Pairing

Sierra Club
www.sierraclub.org

Environmental Action Pairing

Plant a tree in honor of your baby.

journal on

Earth Energy

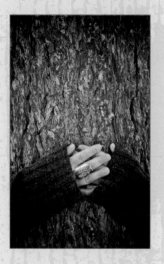

Draw a picture of a nature spot that
reminds you of being grounded, a place
that you can draw from when you need a
quiet place in your mind to visit, perhaps
during your labor.

we are all connected

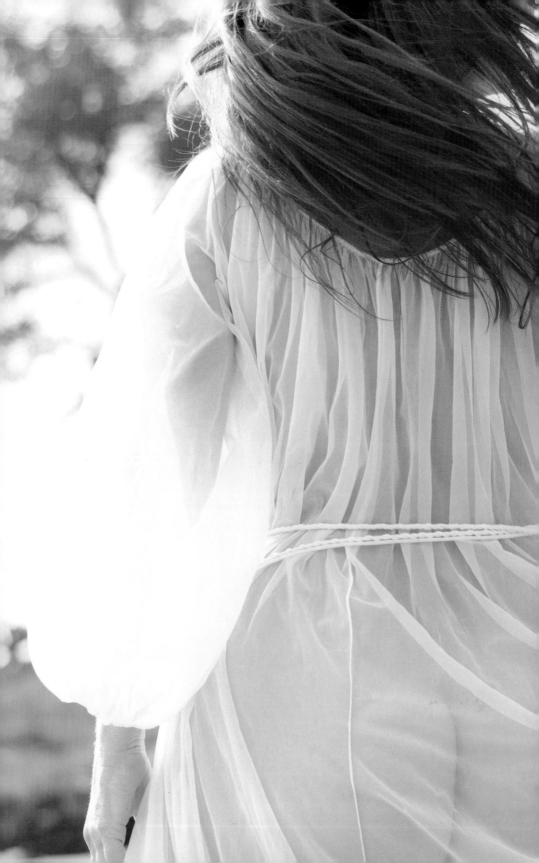

Air Energy

our thoughts are powerful

YOUR BODY ❧

You may be short of breath during this time as your uterus is expanding and pressing on your ribs making it difficult for your lungs to expand. This doesn't allow you much space to breathe. Keep your breath in your conscious awareness so you can begin a regular routine or practice of breath meditation, both to calm your mind and regulate your moods.

YOUR BABY ❧

At twenty-seven weeks, your baby can suck his thumb and his eyes are finally opened. He can sort of respond to light and dark and his kicks should be stronger now that he is living in less fluid. If you are working, now might be the time to really start to dial in your plans for maternity leave. These are hard choices to make, but having the time now to really think it through might provide you more options to stay with your baby as long as possible. This is the week to think!

YOUR SPIRIT ❧

Having a baby is an awesome responsibility, and it can really mess with your mind. The process of a life growing inside a woman's womb is so incredible, it almost seems impossible. This is why creating a breath practice is important to quiet the mind and gain perspective. If you maintain a regular breath practice of deep breathing, this will help with giving birth.

WEEK 27 ❧

The element of air reminds you that the mind has the power to create uplifting and mood-enhancing thought patterns. This topic also speaks to the negative thought patterns that hold us back from reaching our full potential. The pregnant woman has a great challenge to reform her thoughts and create her pregnancy and birth experience just as she wants it. The moment you begin to allow yourself to think negative thoughts (such as, I'm not strong enough or I can't do it), change your thought pattern to uplifting thoughts and see how this practice makes a difference in your pregnancy symptoms. Words and thoughts have tremendous power, choose wisely what passes your lips so you can maintain a stress-free pregnancy.

Reflections

You may be called upon this week to examine your private thoughts about having a baby. Ask yourself some deep questions; are you ready to have a baby and is this what you really want? Do you have reservations about becoming a mother? Are you worried about how this baby will affect your relationship with your partner? Being honest with yourself is the only way to work through any issues that are arising for you. Be honest and process any feelings you are having so you can really step into motherhood clear of mind and heart.

Ideas

- Burn some sage to cleanse your space and mind. If you are struggling with giving yourself positive messages, do this practice every day. Sage is a natural cleanser and can easily shift your mood.

- Try burning incense like sandalwood or Nag Champa to bring your thoughts to a positive space.

- Do regular breath meditations every day, even if only for a few, shortmoments. A regular practice will help you call upon this skill in times of stress and emotional challenges throughout the pregnancy.

Music Pairing

"Bright As Yellow" by The Innocence Mission

journal on

Air Energy

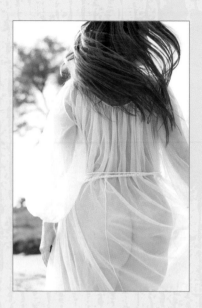

What are the thoughts that have you
up at night in regard to becoming a
mother and giving birth? Lay them
out here in all honesty so that they
can be worked through. Even if they
are irrational ... write them, claim
them, and release them.

our thoughts are powerful

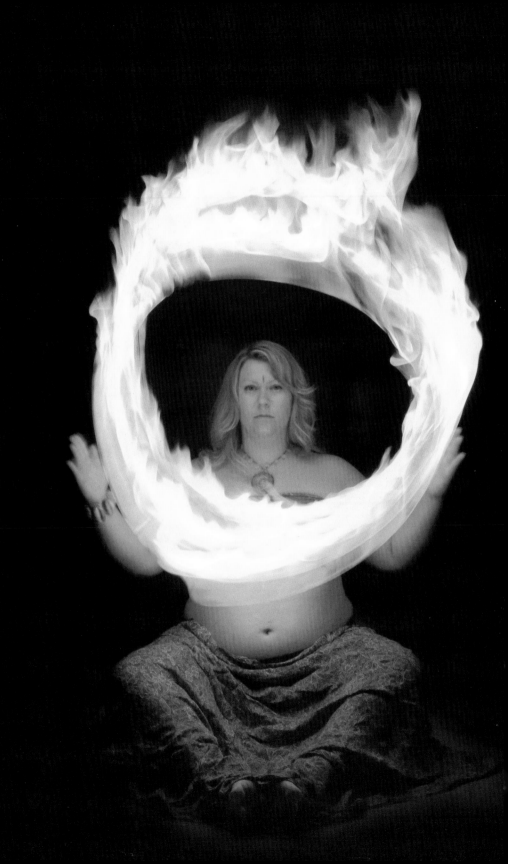

Fire Energy

I can focus my will

to manifest what I want

YOUR BODY ❧

You are entering the third trimester now and hunkering down for the next three months in final prep mode for birth and babe. There are still a few last minutes surprises on the pregnancy train, and one is potential sciatic issues. This is a sharp pain that shoots down the back of your leg starting under your buttocks. It's unpleasant and occurs if the baby is positioned in a certain way. All you can do is rest, ask your partner very kindly for a massage, and ask your baby to move a little. Gathering up your fire energy, your chi, your will to birth your baby takes strength. Rest up now so you are ready to rock when the big day comes.

YOUR BABY ❧

Your baby is settling into his birthing position this week, which hopefully means head down and feet up. Your little sweetie is about two and a half pounds. and is working hard to practice all of his new skills, like blinking and getting into REM sleep patterns. Your baby will have to find the fire inside him when it comes to the birthing day, just like you. He will work just as hard as you will, and needs to have the will, desire, and strength to enter the world and leave your cozy womb. Keep in mind when you are laboring and going through surges, that the two of you are working as one, dynamic team.

YOUR SPIRIT ❧

You are getting closer, Mama! Hang in there and know that the time has come to focus on what you *really* want. There has been a lot of focus up until now on how you are feeling and what is happening in your body, with your baby and your spirit. I have asked you to look deeply at yourself and ask a lot of hard questions. Now is time for action, for making those final decisions about what you want for your birthing experience. This week requires a good look into your heart space to determine what truly lives in there regarding birthing *this* baby at *this* time in your life. You are feeling more ready as the weeks go by, starting to feel Braxton Hicks contractions and the reality of birth is impending—not scary, just coming up. The element of fire is a call to burn away any last fears so you can make room for focused intentions. If you want a natural birth, say it to the universe, write it down, intend it, and then have it! You are all-powerful and came here a gifted person. You are able and if you are willing, you can have exactly what you intend! Live in confidence and life will follow you around like a puppy.

WEEK 28 ☙

Have you ever heard the saying, "Don't play with fire because you're likely to get burned"? It's obviously true, but is used as a poignant metaphor for life. If you engage in reckless behavior, you are likely to get hurt. Fire is a very powerful element and when using it, handle the energy with care. Fire represents our will, passion and intention. The flames of life burn in women and are intended to be intense so we can get those babies out of us. While birthing, many women say they feel a "burning sensation." This feeling is a real-life motivator to push past it to get your baby out and into the world, so use the power of fire with clear intentions and focused will.

Reflections

Fire is a great element to call upon for your birth. However, before you ask this very powerful element for help, you have to *really* know what you want and desire for your experience. Look deep within to determine what you intend and what your true passion is. Be clear so you can have razor sharp focus when it comes to manifesting and birthing your baby into the world. Ask yourself the good questions, such as "Do I want a natural birth and am I committed to that?" "Do I want interventions during the birth, or do I want to intend that nothing extra will be needed?" Watch a flame burn some time, and see the steadiness with which it offers heat and light. Be steady at your birth, be focused, be full of desire and passion, and will it! This may sound like crazy talk to some of you, but it does work, and when you are in labor you will want as many tools as you can fit in your mommy bag to help keep you clear, focused, and determined.

Ideas

- Light a candle everyday on your pregnancy altar. This will help you to stay focused and to *will* your ideal pregnancy into reality. When we use our manifesting skills to let the universe know what we want and we use the power of our intention to get us there, we are far more likely to have a smooth pregnancy and birthing experience.

- Have candles lit at the birth. A flame can become a nice focal point and will remind you of your passion for your baby and your determination to move her into the world with a loving force that only a mother has.

- Ask your sisterhood circle to light candles when you go into labor. This is an extended support system.

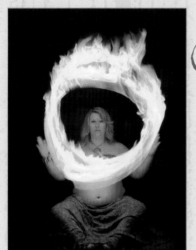

Journal on *Fire Energy*

Are you confident that you know what you want for this pregnancy and birth? If you are not, take the time to get clear and journal about your confusion. When you are ready to really direct your will and intention, the universe will be ready to hear it!

I can focus my will to manifest what I want

Journal on
Fire Energy

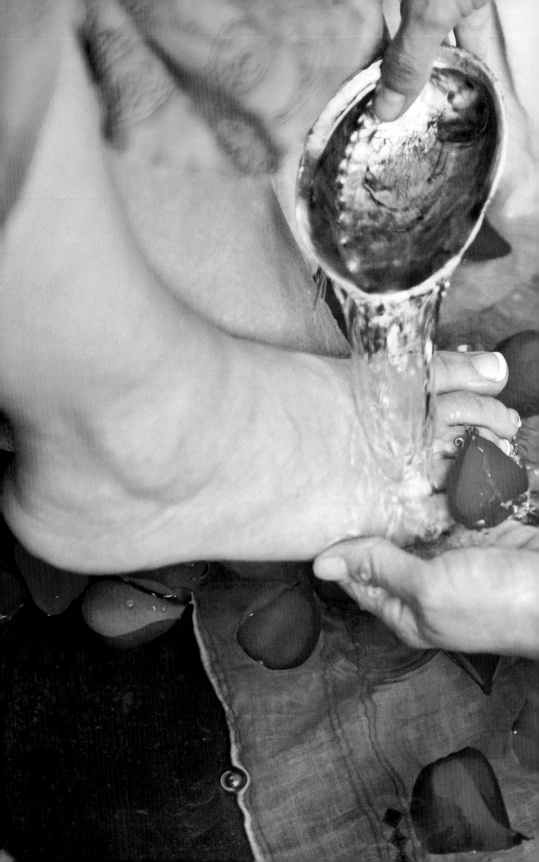

Water Energy

water is woman

embrace the flow

YOUR BODY ☙

Always go to the water! When you have pregnancy aches and pains, submerge yourself in warm waters. It's healing and soothing and reminds us of being a woman. Let your bath become a trusted friend as you spend time with your baby in the water, talking to her and teaching her the ways of woman. You probably have an itchy belly, some swelling, and possible hemorrhoids, so the water is your friend! Remember that all of these symptoms are temporary and magically go away after the baby is born.

YOUR BABY ☙

Your baby lives in water and can breathe water! Did you know that? They are like little amphibians until the cord is cut and they breathe on their own. The buoyancy of water is supportive, warm, and comforting for a baby, just like it offers you comfort when your body aches. Your baby is weighing in at about three pounds now and responds to light and sound.

YOUR spirit ☙

Give yourself the gift of water this week. Spend time close to the ocean, a lake, or a pond or even take a few extra baths. Water is a cleansing element that represents the flow of our every feeling and therefore is the home we should return to when dealing with issues that need to flow out of our lives. Do you ever just go to the beach to sit and look at the ocean? Why do people do this, do you think? It's because the ocean has an energy, a rhythmic flow to it that just comforts us. If we are blessed, like my dear friend Elena (who is one of the photographers of this book), to live in a place like Maui, then we get the bonus of warm, clear ocean waters that feed our souls from the wells of the earth. Why do people like waterfalls? Because their beauty and energy are untouchable, almost magical, and fill a need in us to believe in nature as a healer. Standing under a waterfall, allowing the natural power of that flow to fall upon our heads is an experience like no other. Keep in mind your baby is also living in healing waters and remind yourself this is where to begin to heal if you have any issues that are present during to your pregnancy. Always go to the water!

WEEK 29 ☙

Remember having your period before you got pregnant? Did you ever cramp up and take a nice warm bath to sooth those cramps? Water carries energy that uplifts a woman's body in need, so submerging in a warm tub of water when you are laboring or going through "surges." Whether it's a birthing tub or just your bathtub, this is a natural way to help you through the process of birth. Even if you are planning a hospital birth, you can always begin your laboring at home in the water. You will be surprised at how much this helps you!

Reflections

Water is the most supportive element there is for a woman. Warm waters heal aching bodies, support our bones, and relieve us from the heaviness of life. As I am writing this, I am looking upon my backyard, which has a mini-lake in it. A blue heron arrived, sitting at the edge and waiting for frogs to hop along its path. As I watched this amazing creature walk along the water's edge, thinking about writing on this topic, I was incredibly moved. I wanted to rush over and hug this bird for its inspiration and at the same time, just sit quietly and watch it sink into the depths of the pond, doing what nature intended. Women and water belong together. They are made for each other and they thrive off of one another. Water represents the flow of our emotions and feelings and allows us the space to cry when we need to, bleed with other women, and cleanse our spirit in the holy waters of the sea. Many women choose to have their babies in water because they see the mother wisdom in their baby swimming from the mother's sea to the open waters of life. The transition moves from one natural environment to another that they are used to. This is one of several sacred ways to birth your baby, but it's important to look at the deep wisdom that lives in this approach.

Have you ever seen a woman give birth with dolphins present? When this happens, the most miraculous thing occurs, the dolphins protect the birthing mother and actually support her. When I birthed my last baby River at home underwater, the visual of dolphins was my focal point. I knew that they were a natural part of the birthing world and for some reason, their energy gave me strength and brought calm to my birth.

Ideas

- Let the waters of life support you by gathering water from your favorite space, like the ocean, a lake, or even just an herb-infused bathtub and pour it over your head, committing yourself to being strong for your baby and for birth.
- Try laboring in the tub, even if you are planning a hospital birth.

Website Pairing

Water Birth
www.waterbirth.org

Video Pairing

Ricki Lake and Abby Epstein's documentary *More Business of Being Born*

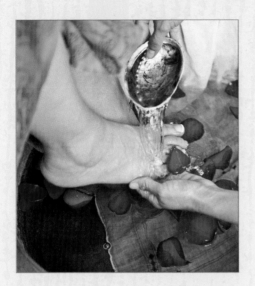

Water Energy

Have you considered laboring and birthing in the water? What are your thoughts on this and are there any feelings relating to this process that you feel you need to cleanse at this time?

water is woman
embrace the flow

journal on

Water
Energy

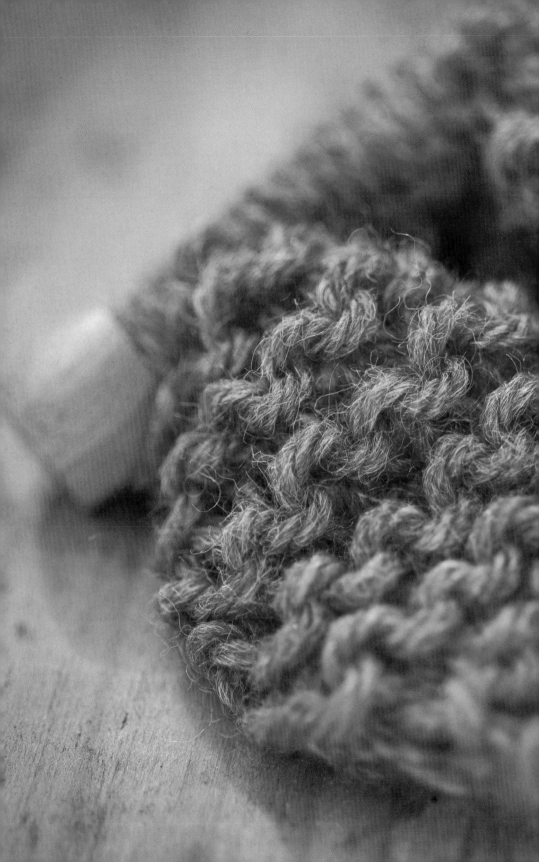

Nesting

gather, cleanse,
knit, and fold

YOUR BODY ℰ∿

You may begin to experience swelling that is not very comfortable. This is a true sign of needing to slow down and put your feet *literally* up—perhaps start knitting those booties! Although your urge will be to go-go-go to get ready for baby, I encourage you to take it day by day at a pace that your body can handle. Also, watch out if you are doing any excessive ice chewing—this is a sign of low iron. If you need an extra boost of iron, check out our iron-rich foods list on page xx. You can supplement with Floradix liquid iron and/or blackstrap molasses.

YOUR BABY ℰ∿

A baby at thirty weeks is starting to see and distinguish light from dark. Pretty cool, huh? She is starting to take up more space in your uterus, and thus your amniotic fluids will be lower. Keep drinking that coconut water! It's great for balancing pH levels and keeping you hydrated and well-nourished. Just as you feel the nesting instincts, so does your baby. She is beginning to settle in now, awaiting her big arrival, and spending these last weeks gaining weight and getting cute!

YOUR SPIRIT ℰ∿

You are likely getting this super-rushed urge to scrub, clean, and organize. This "nesting" instinct is an organic way to begin preparing for your new baby's arrival. You may have the need to create a million lists and feel like you need to buy out every baby store in your town *right now,* but these feelings are merely signals to begin this process— if you go a little slower, you may enjoy these last weeks a little more. Although shopping and decorating is a fun part of being pregnant and preparing for baby, what your baby truly needs is a well-rested mama who is strong of heart and mind and who feels ready to take on mothering. So give yourself some time during this nesting period to make sure *you* feel ready, and don't distract yourself with the stuff. You will actually be surprised how very few things you *really* need to buy. (When they get older, that is another story all together!) Check out the eco-nesting must-haves on page 224 for simple, practical goodies to get you started.

WEEK 30 ☙

First of all, take a deep breath and know that no matter how many times you scrub that floor, it won't get clean enough for the nesting mama. Be aware that nesting is a stepping stone to birthing, and ultimately to holding your baby in your arms—your instincts are prepping you to get ready, not to make you an insane clean freak. If you can slow down and possibly start knitting something for your baby or creating a quilt, this will also serve that purpose of nesting while purposefully slowing you down a little. It's fine and wonderful to get the space ready for baby and something that you really need to do, but do not neglect preparing yourself as well.

Reflections

Talk with your own mother or grandmother about "nesting." Ask them what their experiences were with this when they were pregnant once upon a time. This is a special time that can bring you closer together with your extended family, so try to include them in this process. What grandmother doesn't like to shop for her upcoming grandbaby? Perhaps spend an afternoon out with your own mother purchasing needed items, having lunch, and refreshing your home with the new baby gear.

Ideas

· Emotional nesting: "Mama-nesting" means that you are taking the time to clean out the mental junk that may be hanging out in your emotional basement. Do some emotional housecleaning, releasing fears about becoming a mother and replacing them with trusting your instincts. You can do this by burning a candle and writing all of the emotional things you would like to release on it (buy a seven-day glass jar candle from the Latin food section in the market—they cost around a buck) and then light your candle with the intention of release. Let that sucker burn until it's all gone, maintaining your intention while it's happening. This may take up to seven days, so don't blow it out until it's burned down. (To keep it safe, put it in your bathtub when you leave the house.) After it has burned down, create a new candle and write all your wishes for the new baby, your home, and your and your partner's relationship with her as you create this new family. Let that burn all the way down, knowing at the end you will have willed some deep emotional release to occur and replaced worry with powerful feelings of trust and motherly love.

· Physical nesting

Website Pairing

EcoBaby Planning and Concierge
  Melanie Monroe
  ecobabyplanning.com

Green Nest and Healthy Home Advocates
  Rachel Myers
  greenhugs.net

I went to experts to get you the best, most eco-friendly lists I could; Melanie and Rachel are the best at what they do. So take a gander at these lists to help you in preparing for your new little baby!

ECO-NESTING MUST-HAVES
FROM MELANIE AT ECO BABY PLANNING

· Moby Belly Postpartum Wrap by Moby and Anni Daulter
· Organic mattress or an organic mattress pad, if co-sleeping
· Nook organic crib mattress (unless you co-sleep)
· Oeuf organic crib (unless you co-sleep)
· Organic Cloud and Stars sheets, cloudsandstars.com
· Ultrasonic humidifier/night-light
· Levana Babyview20 video baby monitor
· Baby Planet or Orbit Baby eco-friendly stroller

- aden + anais organic swaddle blankets
- Organic cotton velour sleepsack from Pure Pixie, etsy.com/listing/48959841/eco-friendly-sleep-sack-baby-elephant

  or
- Organic sleepsack from Under the Nile, shop.anthropolobaby.com/Under-the-Nile-Muslin-Organic-Sleep-Sack-UTNSpring3.htm
- Organic wrap sling from Moby or Ergo organic baby carrier
- Phil & Ted's Lobster Chair or Badger Basket wooden high chair
- Sloomb or Fuzzi Bunz cloth diapers or, if using disposables, Bambo Nature diapers or GDiapers
- Reusable flannel baby wipes with a Lionheart Warmies cloth warmer or Nature Baby flushable baby wipes
- A stainless-steel trash can for diapers or The Mother Ease diaper pail, kellyscloset.com/Mother-Ease-Diaper-Pail_p_3936.html
- Earth Mama Angel Baby organic Postpartum Bath Herbs
- For diaper rash: an aloe plant or Angel Baby Bottom Balm
- Argington changing table (converts to a bookshelf)
- Serta organic changing pad
- ABC organic cotton velour changing pad cover
- Gerber organic pre-fold cloth diaper/burp cloths
- Petunia Pickle Bottom organic cotton diaper bag
- The Nose Frida nasal aspirator
- Buzz B battery-operated nail trimmer by Zoli
- The Beaba Babycook
- *Organically Raised: Conscious Cooking for Babies and Toddlers* by Anni Daulter
- Exergen temporal thermometer
- Charlie's laundry soap
- Kate Quinn organic kimonos and infant sacks

- The Spa Baby eco-tub (or just bathe with your baby—it's super fun and easy!)
- The Knottie by Lala's Pequeños
- Baby shampoo and wash by Baby Bear Shop or Erbaviva organic baby wash bag
- Peace sign wooden teether from rocklovepeace
- Organic cotton nursing pillow from Pristine Planet
- Hygeia Enjoy breast pump
- Breastmilk freezer-storage bags or cube trays
- Klean Kanteen or Earthlust stainless steel baby bottles (if you need a bottle at all)
- Bamboobies breast pads
- Motherlove breast cream
- Majamas organic maternity and nursing bras
- Glamourmom nursing tanks
- Moonlight energy-saving night-light
- Svan baby bouncer
- Boon Grass drying rack
- Caldrea Sweet Pea stain remover
- Episencial or Method baby lotion

ECO-CLEANING TIPS
FROM RACHEL AT GREEN HUGS

As a green mama on a budget, I strive to teach people that the things we think we can't live without are actually dangerous products that we should never have been living with in the first place. Chemicals, plastics, and toxins in our everyday products are unfortunate hazards that we need to learn to avoid.

Babies explore the world with hands, feet, and mouths. It is essential that what they touch is free from residue of toxic products—you do not want baby absorbing it through their mouths, skin, and lungs. Think of it this way: you can keep your cabinets and drawers free from products so toxic that if your child got into them that you would have to call 911! If it isn't okay to get into, why would you spread it around your home?

Thankfully, with a little knowledge and armed with a Green Hugs-approved product list, your nest can be a safe haven for health and comfort, all wrapped up in a budget-friendly package! Compiled with love of family and a disdain for chemicals, here is a list of cleaning must-have's that will keep your family safe and your nest sparkling!

GREEN HUGS CLEANING ESSENTIALS

- Clean well: As far as hand-sanitizing spray, foaming hand soap, and wipes go, every green mama knows they are a staple at changing stations and in diaper bags everywhere! Unfortunately, most anti-bacterials contain Triclosan, a nasty biocide that should be kept out of your nest. Just replacing your sprays, soaps, and wipes with the Clean Well line takes this chemical out of your home. Buy the great smelling line at binibirth.com/default.asp.

- Earthworm family-safe cleaning products: From floors to counters to an odor-eliminating spray, Earthworm products stand out for safety and affordability. Earthworm uses natural, enzyme-based sprays that break down organic materials. They leave your home safely clean and deodorized.

- Biokleen laundry detergent: Phosphate- and chlorine-free, Biokleen detergent keeps clothes clean and soft without the use of harsh chemicals. It is my favorite detergent and is cloth-diaper safe. They also carry Bac-Out stain and odor eliminator, which is a great pre-treatment for your cloth diapers. biokleenhome.com

- Rockin Green Soap: RGS is a fantastic mom-made laundry detergent that smells delicious, is cloth-diaper safe, and works like a charm. It is a cult favorite and can be used with confidence for your entire family's laundry. From Bare Naked Babies to Smashing Watermelons, the all-natural scents can't be beat! www.rockingreen soap.com

- Ecover dishwasher tablets: Ecover dishwasher tablets are phosphate-free and actually work at getting your dishes clean and sparkling. It is an affordable and safe line. I also recommend their laundry stain remover and fabric softener. www.ecover.com

For the true Do-It-Yourself Mama, make your own green cleaning products. The ratio for using vinegar to clean is usually one cup of vinegar to two cups of water. For heavier cleaning, I use straight vinegar. The strong vinegar smell will dissipate when it dries. Use a glass spray bottle when mixing your own spray cleaners.

There are four main components to cleaning:

- Bleaching: baking soda or lemon
- Disinfecting: Vinegar
- Killing germs: Lemon or essential oils like tea tree oil
- Conditioning wood or leather: olive oil

TOILET BOMBS

Add vinegar and baking soda to your toilet bowl. Watch it bubble up, don't flush and leave overnight to clean and disinfect. The next morning use a bowl brush to swipe it down and then flush!

FURNITURE POLISH

½ teaspoon oil, such as olive

¼ cup vinegar or fresh lemon juice

Mix the ingredients in a glass jar. Dab a soft rag into the solution and wipe onto wood surfaces. Cover the glass jar and store indefinitely.

ALL-PURPOSE GREEN AND CLEAN SPRAY

Mix one teaspoon Castile soap or plant-based liquid soap and three tablespoons distilled white vinegar with two cups of water in a spray bottle and shake.

Green Hugs, Rachel Myers

BIRTH NESTING

If you are having a home birth, don't forget to order your birth kit, and if you are having a birth-center or hospital birth, start by buying the right bag for you to take with you and pack your focal point art work first thing!

Just like packing for a weekend away, take the necessities.
The things that make you feel like *you*!

- A picture ID (driver's license or other ID)
- Your insurance card, and any hospital paperwork you need
- Your birth plan, if you have one
- Eyeglasses and/or contacts
- Toiletries: Toothbrush and toothpaste, lip balm, deodorant, a brush and comb, a hair band or barrettes, and makeup, if you wear it
- Sanitary pads (try Glad Rags)
- Bathrobe
- Sleeveless, loose nightgowns
- Warm socks or slippers
- Camera and/or video camera
- Call list to announce the event to friends and family
- Cell-phone charger
- Comfy nursing bras (like Majamas and I in the Oven) and soft, re-usable breast pads
- Organic maternity underwear (Carriwell.com)
- This journal and pen to record your memories and feelings of the experience while they're fresh and you have a few quiet minutes
- A yummy receiving blanket or organic swaddle blanket
- Going-home outfit with hat

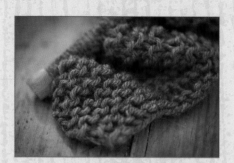

journal on

Nesting

Write about your release ritual and whether or not you feel "mother-nested" now. Also use this space to make those lists!

gather, cleanse, knit, and fold

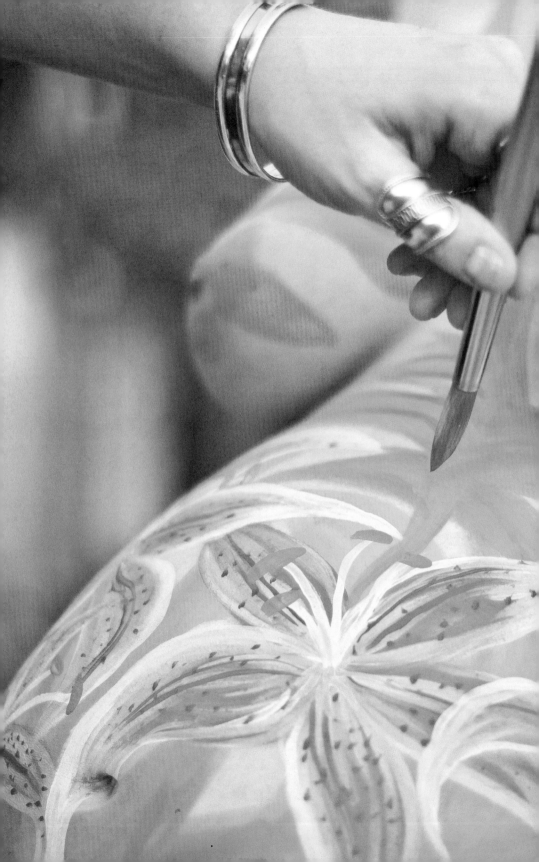

Adornment

*decorate your belly
with pride, love, and humility*

YOUR BODY ⟡

Well you probably have to pee every second, and your belly is so big that it probably feels uncomfortable to lie on your side at night. This is where the delicious body pillow comes to the rescue. I recommend that you buy one—they are amazing for supporting you under your belly and in between your legs, and this will help you sleep. Remember in the beginning when you needed a *ton* of sleep so the baby could do that very early and important growing? Well at the end of a pregnancy you also need a lot of rest so that you can build up strength to be prepared to go into the birth full of energy. Keep your fluids up because your body is producing blood cells like crazy, and you need to maintain your increased blood volume. Try drinking straight coconut water to increase your alkaline levels and keep your waters plentiful.

YOUR BABY ⟡

A baby at thirty-one weeks is about three and a half pounds and is gaining about a half-pound or so a week until the big day. The kicks start to feel more like swimming and squirming, as she tries to make room and gets nice and plump over these next few weeks. Introduce your baby to your sisterhood tribe, one by one. Your baby can hear and feel, and should know who will be there to support her as she transitions from the coziness of your womb into the arms of her tribe. Who are the women who are there to hold and comfort her as she stretches her little body into the big open world?

YOUR SPIRIT ⟡

You are entering the waiting period now, and it's time to release anxiety and allow those around you to fill you up with their sister strength so that you have a surplus of energy to pull from while birthing the baby. Although only you can birth your baby, you need the support and love of your tribe around you, cheering you on and honoring your courage. Giving birth is an act of bravery and complete trust in the universe, and in our moments of fear and worry, it can be hard to remember that. We need others around us to remind us. Perhaps write this mantra on a piece of paper and tape it to your bathroom mirror: "I am the strength of all women who have ever birthed a baby and I am ready to join that tribe." Having affirmations around the house feeds your subconscious and allows you to dig deep when you really need to.

WEEK 31 ☙

What is adornment and why should you do it? As you can see from the beautiful image Elena captured, adorning your big, round belly with either paint, henna, or beautiful jewels are just a few ways to celebrate that beautiful round glowing belly of yours. This is not done, however, just for the sake of beautifying. While that *is* a perk, adornment also marks the transition from hanging out being pregnant to readying yourself to give birth. Adornment is a sacred ritual for a woman and should be presented to her as a gift. Many women have belly-casting parties accompanied by a small gathering of sisters in a circle who bless and adorn the new mother. These circles are valuable because they are designed to honor you and bow to you in reverence as you create life and are weaved into the fabric of womanhood by this awesome act of courage.

Reflections

Reflect on how you feel about others hosting an honoring circle for you. Are you comfortable with this type of interaction or does it make you feel embarrassed or shy? This next part is *not* for you! This next paragraph is meant for your best girlfriend, so go ahead and give her your *Sacred Pregnancy* book for a few moments so *she* can glean some ideas for adorning her sister.

Ideas

Adornment ritual: This is a gathering that is *just* for mom, not for baby, and as such needs to have her in mind. The mother-to-be should not do any work for this special night and needs to allow herself to be fully given to. The idea is to have her sisters gather in a loving circle to help support her as she prepares to birth her child. The mother-to-be should be showered with love, goodies, and strength and given a power necklace to help her through the last phase of her pregnancy and lend her strength for the birth.

1. Send out special invites to the mother-to-be's tribe of sisters who are dedicated to being a part of her birthing support team.

2. Before the guest of honor arrives, decorate a space for her with comfy pillows, rose petals, warm-water foot soaks, and decadent treats, such as raw chocolate. Have lotions for foot rubs and all the supplies to either do a belly-cast project or a painting on her belly.

3. Ask each woman coming to bring the mother a bead to string together a power necklace with the support of her tribe. It may also be nice to ask each woman attending to bring her a small gift just for her, like new jammies, slippers, books, journals, or a post-pregnancy care package.

4. Create a flower crown for the mother-to-be to wear throughout the party.

5. After all the women have gathered, ask the guest of honor to sit in her special spot and then go around the circle lighting candles of blessings for her as she prepares for birth. Make sure that these blessings speak to this particular mother's strengths and ability to birth with confidence and ease.

6. Soak her feet in warm sea salt and essential-oiled water, then have two to three women massage her feet and legs with lotion.

7. Each woman should offer the mother her "power bead" and one person should be in charge of stringing these together for her. While the mother is receiving these beads, have another sister brush her hair. The idea is to have this mother completely bathed in the love of her sisters, as she prepares for this ultimate rite of passage.

8. Don't forget to massage her aching feet and legs.

9. Either do a belly cast or a belly painting to close out the evening.

Website Pairing

Belly Vita (Belly Castings)
www.bellyvita.com

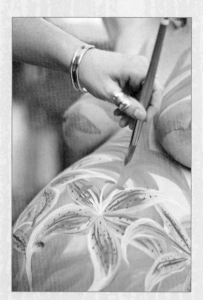

Adornment

What was it like to be nurtured by your tribe of women? Do you feel full of their positive juju after the ritual? Write about the power necklace.

decorate your belly with pride, love, and humility

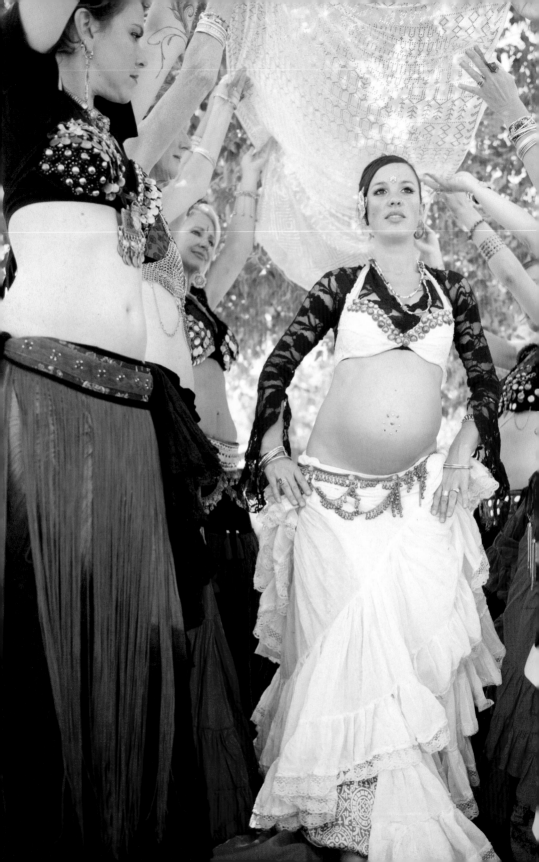

Blessingway

go to the bowl with your tribe,
for your baby

YOUR BODY ◠

You are in the home stretch now and feeling it! You have to pee every ten minutes and you may feel light-headed from time to time, almost like you might faint. During these last weeks, your blood tends to pool in the lower limbs, resulting in low cranial blood pressure that makes you feel dizzy.

YOUR BABY ◠

Your baby at thirty-two weeks is weighing in at around four and a half pounds and may be turning his body to get into the birthing position (with his head down), which means he is pushing down on your abdomen like never before. This can make you feel uncomfortable and like you are ready to have the baby at any given moment. In these final weeks, the baby's lungs are in still developing. Don't worry if you don't feel as many kicks as before—there simply is not as much room in there! The skeleton is developed and bones are there, but start to harden later.

YOUR SPIRIT ◠

Taking time to honor and thank your baby for coming to you is a great way to prepare for her arrival. Allow any feelings of worry or anxiety about the upcoming birth to flow through you, acknowledging them and then releasing them as you move into deep appreciation and excitement. The more joy you infuse into your pregnancy, the easier the birth will be and the smoother the transition into motherhood.

WEEK 32 ◠

Traditionally, folks have what they call *baby showers* for the mom and baby in which they play baby-related games and give a bunch of gifts to the mother for the baby. We have already had a lovely celebration for you and talked about the adornment rituals that can be done to honor you as the mother, but what should you do for the baby if you want to add in a spiritual component to the process? You could host a *blessing-*

way instead of a baby shower. This process honors the family and can include everyone, including younger siblings. This is a ceremony in which people bless the *way* of the baby and the mother as Mama readies herself to birth her baby into existence.

Reflections

What if you want to do these non-traditional ceremonies or rituals, but your partner, and/or family, does not support you in these efforts? These are important questions, as they bring forth real-life situations that may stress you out and leave you feeling isolated and alone.

Ideas

There are many ways to host a blessingway, and many ways to explore this type of celebration.

GOING TO THE BOWL

1. Ask each person coming to the blessingway to bring a bead for the baby, so you can make her a similar necklace to the one you have now from the adornment ritual.

2. Set up a nice circle space with pillows on the floor and a birthing altar in the center with candles, goddess figures, herbs, flowers, and a large bowl filled with sea salt.

3. You may also want to ask everyone to bring a dish to share so that you are not doing a ton of cooking.

4. Sit in a circle and place the salt bowl in front of whoever wants to start the ritual. Ask each person to offer a blessing to the family and the baby and add to the bowl natural goodies, such as essential oils, flower petals, sugars, and herbs. As each person takes a turn doing this, offering a blessing, adding in some herbs and adding in her intentions, the bowl of salts starts to be infused with yummy smells and loving wishes.

5. After each person takes his turn, he should offer their bead to the family.

6. You may want to ask someone to be in charge of crafting a little necklace out of the beads for you.

7. After everyone has "gone to the bowl," you will hand each person a plain, glass Mason jar and ask them to fill it up with some salts that they will take with them.

8. When the mother goes into labor, and they are notified, they are asked to use the salts in their own bath to cleanse in all the loving intentions sent out to the family as a way to be connected to the birth from afar.

9. It is also nice to offer the family gifts for the baby at this celebration, and perhaps have them take a look at a wish list in order to get that planned.

Great Book Pairing (for more ideas)

Mother Rising: The Blessingway Journey into Motherhood by Yana Cortlund, Barb Lucke, and Donna Miller Watelet

Herb Pairing

Mountain Rose Herbs
  www.mountianroseherbs.com

Blessingway

Who attended your blessingway, and what were the special moments about it that you would like to remember to pass down to your child? Perhaps have them write a little blessing here for the baby to hear later.

go to the bowl with your tribe, for your baby

journal on
Blessingway

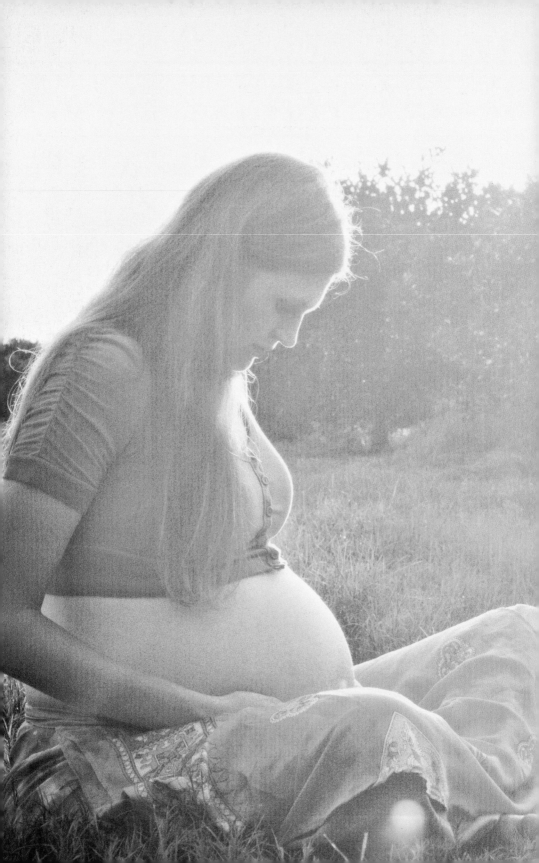

Naming Ceremony

names fulfill destinies

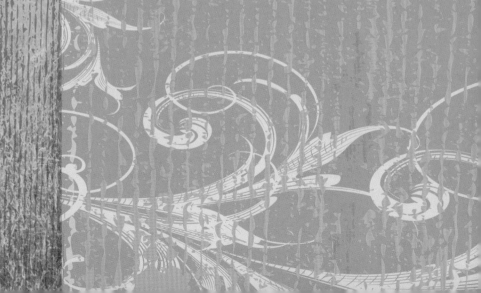

YOUR BODY ⌒

As your belly grows nice and big, other things start to happen within. Your fingers, hands, and wrists may start to feel tingling and numbness. It's normal, so don't freak out—and it's only temporary. It's tough to sleep, so make sure you are using the body pillow and drinking a lot of fluids in the day, slowing down at night so you can halt the number of trips to the bathroom during the night. Distract yourself from these body aches by starting to dream your baby's name into existence.

YOUR BABY ⌒

Your baby at thirty-three weeks is getting big weighing in at around four pounds. Now that your baby is moving and shaking in your baby oven all the time and the due date is coming near, your talking with the baby has likely increased. So what are you calling your belly baby? Sweetie, baby, cutie? These are the first words your baby hears and is likely starting to respond to your chatting, so make your nicknames for your belly baby calm, relaxed, and filled with love. From now on, your baby is just gaining weight, getting pink, and finishing up the development of all his cute details. Your baby's brain grows so rapidly during this week that his head will increase a quarter of an inch this week.

YOUR SPIRIT ⌒

Choosing a name for baby makes this whole thing real. It personalizes it, and gives it life. Heck, you can even go buy that monogrammed hooded baby towel if you have a name all picked out. If you find yourself avoiding choosing names or cannot settle on one, consider what might be holding you back. It could be a sign that you are just not ready for the baby to come and naming him or her brings her that much closer to your arms and the reality that soon you *will* be holding and caring for your new baby. If this is the case, just take notice of it, thank these fears, and release them into the cooling waters of the universe. Know that the choosing of a name *does* make it more real, but it also makes him more a part of your family. As the great poet Rumi said, "Our children are not ours, but they come through us. We do not own them, we guide them." Giving your child a name starts the process of guiding him, and only you have been charged with this task with this baby. How cool is that?

WEEK 33 ☙

What is in a name? It's funny that we have so many baby books with a bunch of names in them, as if we could flip through them to find our child's identity. A name is personal, it's political, it's spiritual, it's artistic, and it's identifying. It's so much fun to name your child, and it's a great time to start really honing in on how and what you will name your baby. What is your relationship with your own name? Do you like it or have you always felt like you wanted to be named something else? Sometimes I meet someone whose name just does not fit them. Has that ever happened to you? Your baby has come to you and your partner for a specific life lesson, and as much as you handle his little body and spirit with care, be careful with his destiny and the name your choose. This is the password to his life path—make it a good one!

Reflections

In many cultures, before they name the child, they wait until the baby is born, until they have met the child, meditated on the matter, and asked the universe for divine inspiration. Others sit under trees and ask for the baby's song to come to them, and in that they find the name. We asked our children to help name our other kids, and we also wanted each child to have a name that fit him or her, a name that offered a pathway to who he or she is meant to be in the world. A person's name is something he hears more than any other word in his lifetime, and it's the essence of who he is and what he is to become. Choose a name with purpose, intention, and meaning. A person's name carries energy and as such should be given with care and after thoughtful meditation.

NAMING STORY

My daughter Lotus came to me in a dream, about one year before I was pregnant with her. She told me she was coming, that her name is Lotus, and that I should start preparing for her. I told my boyfriend, now husband, and he was shocked. Throughout the next year, Lotus would often visit my dreams and give me little updates as to when she was going to arrive.

Ideas

· Meditate and ask the universe to offer some guidance on the naming process.

· Take a look back in your family tree to determine some old family names and their meanings that you had not known before and perhaps adopt a hybrid of one of those.

· My husband and I combined our last name—his was Walter and mine was Dauley, so we made up "Daulter," to give our children only one last name. We went to court and changed our names; now we are the only Daulters that I know of. We both identify so much with our last name as Daulter that we can hardly remember our other last names.

· Consider names from stories that having meaning to you and your partner or from poems, past heroines, ancestors, culture, nature, or something the universe just hands right to you.

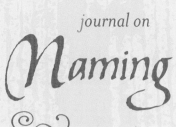

journal on

Naming

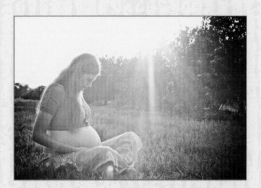

What are your lists of names for both a boy and a girl? What are the meanings of the names and why have you chosen them?

names fulfill destinies

journal on

Naming

Visualization:
Your Perfect Birth

create your own birth experience

YOUR BODY ❧

Although you are feeling pretty big by now, you still have some room to grow. Even though you may not be as hungry as you were in the beginning, having more frequent snacks throughout the day is often better than large meals, and can keep your last bit of growing minimal. Your baby is pushing on your bladder and you may have more frequent urination. It is also normal during this week to start feeling surges, which are your body's way of starting to prepare you for the actual birth. This is like the first phase and does not have pain attached to it, just a tightening feeling that comes and goes. Sleeping may also become more difficult. I always needed that body pillow behind my back, in between my legs, and under my belly to balance out all the weight and to truly feel comfortable. All of these are healthy signs, as it really begins to signal your time is coming closer and your baby will be in your arms soon.

YOUR BABY ❧

A baby at thirty-four weeks is very close to being born and is pretty big, weighing in at just over four pounds, although you may not birth him for another six to eight weeks. Babies continue to put on weight and are now just putting the finishing touches on themselves. The baby is most likely in position, head down and getting prepared to come into the world. Ask your midwife or doctor to check this if you are interested, as a midwife can try to help you turn the baby to avoid a breech-birth situation, should your baby's head not be down.

YOUR SPIRIT ❧

If you do not have a fully formulated birth plan, now is the time to pull it together. This week is a time to start visualizing the way you want this birth to manifest itself. Who do you want to be present? What will you do during your surges, and who will be there reminding you to stay calm and focused, to breathe and relax into each surge? You may be feeling both excitement and nervousness as the due date approaches, but this is the time for grounding and centeredness. Get clear on what you want and start making a plan to birth that into existence.

WEEK 34 ⚬〰

Your mind has tremendous power. If you are able to train your mind to imagine the perfect birth scene for yourself, you are far more likely to be able to form the birth experience that you want. This can include having a painless birth, short labor, and a healthy baby at the end of it all. If you do not have much practice with visualization, take time to research a little bit about it, as it truly can serve as a wonderful tool for you during the birthing process. You may want to investigate hypbirth meditations to help you with this.

Reflections

Do some meditating on how you want the birth experience to go. Who is there? What does it look like? Sound like? Smell like? Answer these questions in the form of a visualization narrative for yourself that you will be able to replay time and time again in your mind until it becomes second nature to you.

Here is a short example of a lovely visualization for the birthing mama.

> *Picture yourself in warm water, with your favorite soft music playing in the background, your loved ones all surrounding you, candles lit, and your belly bursting with life. You know that you are getting so close to meeting your baby for the first time, and you are excited and confident. The sun is going down and the soft glow of the sunset is upon your cheek. You look outside to see some wild flowers growing in your garden. The colors are vibrant and the flowers look full of life. You are holding your belly, talking to your baby, knowing that you will be able to hold and kiss your newborn very soon. You notice each surge as it comes and goes, and you welcome each one, as you know it brings you closer and closer to meeting your baby. You breathe in and out with each surge, releasing your tension into each one. You know that there is something amazing about what you are doing and something familiar about it. You realize that you are a part of the sisterhood community of women who have birthed before you, and who are now standing in*

their power for you. In a short while, you will step over that threshold into motherhood and will know that you are a part of the tribe. You feel strong and confident, and know that you can do it. Remember, you can birth your baby. You are strong and powerful and you know inherently how to do this. Stand in your power and welcome your brand new healthy child into your clan.

Ideas

- Write down exactly how you want your birth to go. This will become your manifestation tool over the next few weeks while you are mentally and emotionally preparing to give birth.

- Choose a couple of words as a mantra for you during birth that will immediately take you to your "perfect birth" scene.

Book Pairing

The Creative Visualization Workbook, Second Edition by Shakti Gawain

Audio Pairing

Hypbirth Series (hypbirth.com/ordering.html)
  These CDs are amazing!

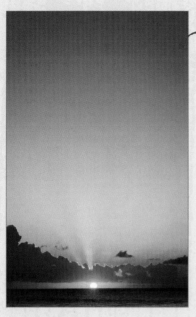

journal on

Visualion:

Your Perfect Birth

Take time to write down your own visualization scene to manifest your perfect birth. Be specific and speak to every aspect of this sacred process and how you want it to go. Use your power to create the birth you want!

create your own birth experience

Visualization:
Your Perfect Birth

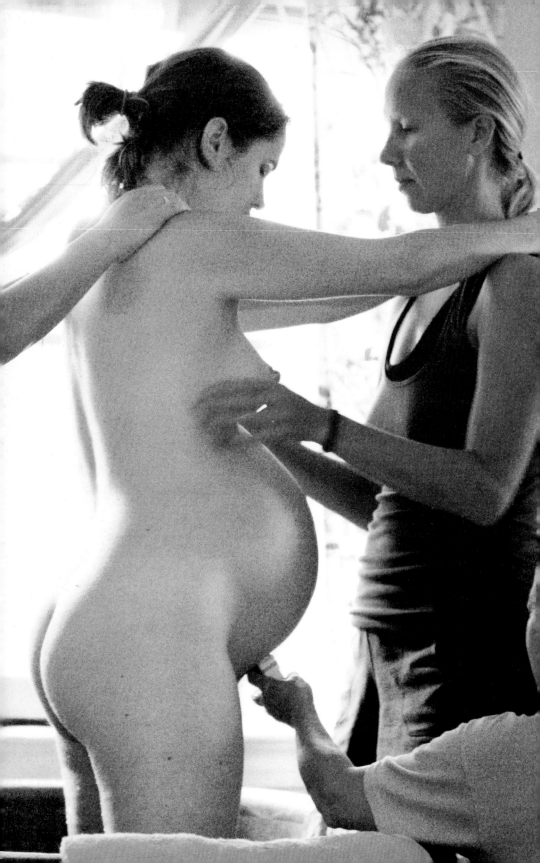

Empowerment

*you are all woman and
that means all-powerful*

YOUR BODY ⌒

This week, focus on finding your voice and breathing. As you near your due date, breathwork practice is critical and becoming empowered enough to advocate for yourself will require using that mother-voice of yours. If you are not used to that, it could be hard for you to do. As you are getting pretty big now, you might also find breathing difficult and discover that huge meals are too much for you. Eating smaller, more frequent meals may work better for you.

YOUR BABY ⌒

At thirty-five weeks, your baby is a baby, pretty plump, and full of cuteness, but still putting on the pounds. At this point, your baby is growing about an ounce a day, which is a lot, and the lungs are almost fully developed. If you don't have a car seat, now might be the time to grab that hot-ticket item. Get it set up and practice playing with it if you do not know how they work. It's is also fun to have the car seat in the car because it makes the baby's pending arrival seem more real.

YOUR SPIRIT ⌒

To be empowered is to be uplifted and supported, and at this point in the pregnancy game, you need to down gallons of that Kool-Aid so that you are ready to jump into the deep end of your birthing pool without a floaty. When you are practicing breathing try this birth breath:

1. When you breathe in, say in your mind, "I am powerful."

2. When you breath out, say out loud, "I can do it."

It's important to say affirmations and mantras out loud because you need to practice hearing your voice claim your power. You are entitled to your own birth power, but you will only be able to find what you need in your own toolbox. Use this breath exercise in birth as well if you find it helpful.

Do you feel empowered and ready to birth your baby? Do you feel like your birthing team has come together to help lift you up in ways that make you feel like you really can do it? Being empowered to birth your baby is not the traditional model of care in the modern birthing world in this country. In fact, it's quite the opposite. Most women feel like they do not know what they are doing, are afraid, and, because of the horror stories they have heard, shy away from feeling that they can birth naturally without drug interventions. Being empowered means knowing your rights—knowing your body, your spirit, and your baby and trusting that all of these components will work harmoniously with one another on the day of the birth. It's also allowing others to help you when you need it and expressing your needs and desires by putting a flexible birthing plan in place. So empower yourself to find your "birth voice" and add your song to the chorus of women who have sung this tune for many moons before you.

Reflections

Have you always been able to advocate for yourself when you need to? If you are not the type of person who feels like you will be able to speak up for what you want and need at your birth, then make sure to look deeper at this issue and practice using your voice to express your needs. You may want to consider hiring a doula to help support and advocate for you. What messages did you get growing up around being vocal about your needs? If you want a doula, but don't have one yet, start interviewing them now. Call Binibirth to discuss your options if you do not know where to start this process; Ana Paula is an amazing doula and can help guide you in finding the right match.

Using your voice is a huge part of being empowered. Since we are focusing on your breathwork this week, add in an empowering mantra. When practicing your breathwork say, "I am strong and empowered" with each breath. Simple and short mantras are great when doing patterned breathwork and a nice way to plant a new message in your unconscious mind so that it is easy to pull back up into your conscious mind during the birthing process.

A NOTE ON EMPOWERMENT
FROM MIDWIFE KATIE MCCALL

To be a midwife is to be with women. Every culture and every era has had its wise woman, its sage femme, its crone, its priestess. These women are the lamps that light the path for the women in their community. They show the way to go: spiritually, emotionally, psychologically, and sometimes even physically. They are moved to do so by a divine calling and recognized in their work by the women in their community.

Midwife is not synonymous with woman-doctor. While doctors are instrumental in the lives of a community's women, doctors are mechanics of biology and anatomy. They are the astronomers of anatomy and the explorers of pathology. Their playing field is the physical realm; the human body is their instrument.

Midwifery is not deformed obstetrics and neither is obstetrics an injured form of midwifery. Midwifery and obstetrics are unique and separate, yet can support one another as harmoniously as a mother and father in a household setting.

Midwives are mothers. Even if they have no children of their own, midwives mother the mothers they serve. Their job is to work themselves out of a job by empowering mothers to take the reigns in their own sexual, relational, and birthing processes. In this way, the women in a community can only be as healthy and empowered as their midwives are.

To be a midwife is to be with women. It is to be with them when they cry with the loss of a baby, to hold space for them when they work through finding safety from a batterer, to laugh when they share their child's first steps, to listen when they process birth fears or menopause frustrations, to provide non-judgment when they speak out about sexual dysfunction and find their place within it, or to offer kindness and wisdom and compassion when they are hurting or working hard.

To be a midwife is not simply the act of catching a baby. Catching a baby is one of midwifery's greatest honors—but if you spend enough time with a midwife, she will tell you it is the least complex part of her calling. A midwife's highest honor is to discover that women who were once dependent on her no longer need her ... just like any other mother.

Ideas

- Write a birth manifesto! Make a few vows to yourself.

- Do some *birth art* and create a collage of images that represent being empowered to you. Place this piece of art on your birth altar, and consider having it at the birth. Save this and frame it for your child. Passing along empowerment to your child is worth doing.

- Make or buy an empowerment necklace to wear at the birth. This will be a physical reminder that you can do it and are empowered enough to birth your baby. Some women like to wear rose quartz because it represents love; some like a cowry shell to represent opening your body to birth; some like a tiger's eye for protection; even your baby's birth stone would be a nice choice.

Movie Pairing

Every Mother Counts documentary by Christy Turlington

Music Pairing

"I Am the Water" by Aradhana Silvermoon

journal on

Empowerment

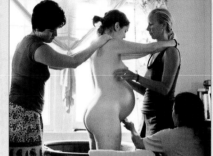

Write down your birth mantra so
that you know what it is and what
worked for you when you are
practicing your birth breathing.

you are all woman and that means all-powerful

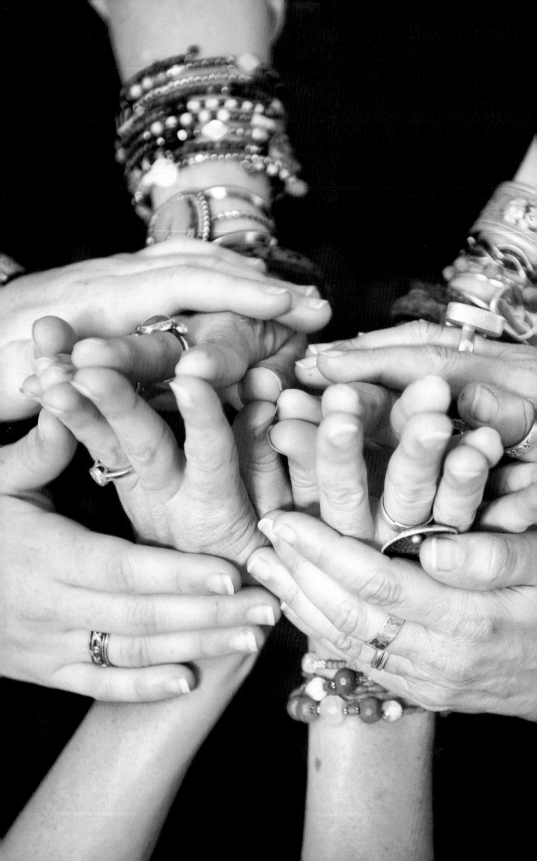

Sisterhood

gather your tribe

YOUR BODY ⟍

The time is near and your body knows it. Even if you are not mentally ready yet, your body is the driving force here—so give it what it asks for! Plenty of good, healthy power foods, rest, and relaxation. Thirty-six weeks is always the time when I would meet with my midwives for that "talk" about the birth: the talk to make sure all of my affairs were in order and that I had all I needed for the birth. It is finally the time to put your feet up and really go over that birthing plan in detail and even if your birth plan goes up in a puff of smoke, being focused and prepped is always a good idea.

YOUR BABY ⟍

At the end of this week, your baby will be considered full term and is already about six pounds and about eighteen inches long. What this means in real-life is that anytime your baby decides to come between now and forty-two to forty-three weeks will likely result in a nice plump and healthy babe. From now until your baby does join you will just be spent packing on the pounds.

YOUR SPIRIT ⟍

At this point there are so many feelings swimming around, it's diffi-cult to bring any of them into focus. This is the time to gather your tribe, your sisters, the women in your life, and "go to the bowl." *(See Week 32, Blessingway, on page 241.)* My midwife held monthly new moon circles where there was a huge bowl in the center filled with sacred salts and several women would come, sit around the bowl, explore their feelings on the topic of the month, and add their blessings to the bowl. I adopted that ritual with my tribe and you can too.

As you are preparing to birth your baby, you need the support of women around you and to be held in their strength as you prepare for your rite of passage into motherhood. If you are having a home birth, gather your birthing supplies in a big basket to keep them orga-nized and make sure your house is stocked with restorative foods like the makings for a nice kale soup and some juices. Talk to your doula or other support women and get your plans in order to determine who will start the phone tree for when you need your tribe to gather, light candles, and sing your praises as you pull your deepest strength together in preparation for the glorious event. If you are having a birth-center birth or delivering in a hospital, gather your things and be ready to go. You can designate someone to try to create a comfortable space for you outside of your home by bringing music, candles, pictures, and objects that may help you keep focused like a birthing woman statue of some sort (see Resources on page 321 for places to buy).

WEEK 36 ⌒

Birth is a sacred practice that only women can experience and this miracle, in many cultures, has been supported by a woman's tribe—her sisters, her friends, her female relatives, her circle. As the mystery of the baby forms in a woman's womb, her sisters can help her to decipher the flow of emotion and the physical transformations that come with the many phases of her pregnancy. It is so valuable to provide sacred support for a woman in her space of transitioning into motherhood and to help her join with her higher female self, her power as a creator of life.

Reflections

Make a list of your own tribe of women. Who do you trust to have in your circle to support you, not only through this pregnancy, but through motherhood? Spend some time with the women in your circle, and ask them the questions that you have in your heart about this very sacred rite of passage. Let them support and honor you through this process.

You may want to take time to connect with your own mother, and revisit the stories of your own birth. This action can help you begin your own birthing process fresh and filled with your own her-story of how you came into the world through your female lineage. Remember that even if you are physically alone, you have other women in the world who are spiritually connected to you, who care and who want you to have a beautiful birthing experience. If you feel isolated and alone and do not feel as though you have a sisterhood to turn to, build one or connect with an existing one. Don't forget that you can join the online Sacred Pregnancy community of women for support and look for a Sacred Pregnancy circle in your area. You can also find others that may work for you, such as Binibirth. I have said this before, but it's worth repeating: you are part of the collective circle of women and by birthright, you are entitled to a place in this sacred tribe.

Ideas

- A simple idea is to make a lunch date with a special woman in your life and to bask in the energy of the divine female.

- Learn about how you came into the world. Talk to your own mother about her experience when you were born. If you are unable to do that, try talking with another relative that could have been there at the time, just to gain some interpersonal perspective.

- Invite several women over for a special circle where you are honored and showered as you step into the place of birthing. (See Week 31, Adornment, on page 233 for more specifics.)

- Have a good, old-fashioned sleepover, like the ones you used to have as a teenager. Invite some of your girls over for movies, popcorn, chocolate ice cream, and cozy connection.

- Take the time to create your birth call tree, a phone list of all those you want to know you are in labor, and decide whether or not you want any of your sisterhood tribe at the birth to support you. If you do not have any one you feel could do that, consider hiring a doula to be present with you at the birth.

- Try connecting to Binibirth, a community of supportive birthing professionals and doulas, at binibirth.com.

Book Pairing

The Red Tent by Anita Diamant and the Rent Tent Movement

Website Pairing

Mystic Mama

www.mysticmamma.com

Fun Outing Pairing

Go see *Motherhood, the Musical!*

journal on

Sisterhood

Take time to journal what you
may have discovered about the
time when you were born and
how that affects you today. What
might you want to explore more
deeply to prepare you for this
birthing experience and who is
your sisterhood? Name them!

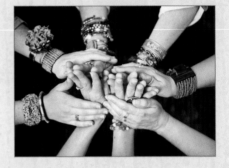

gather your tribe

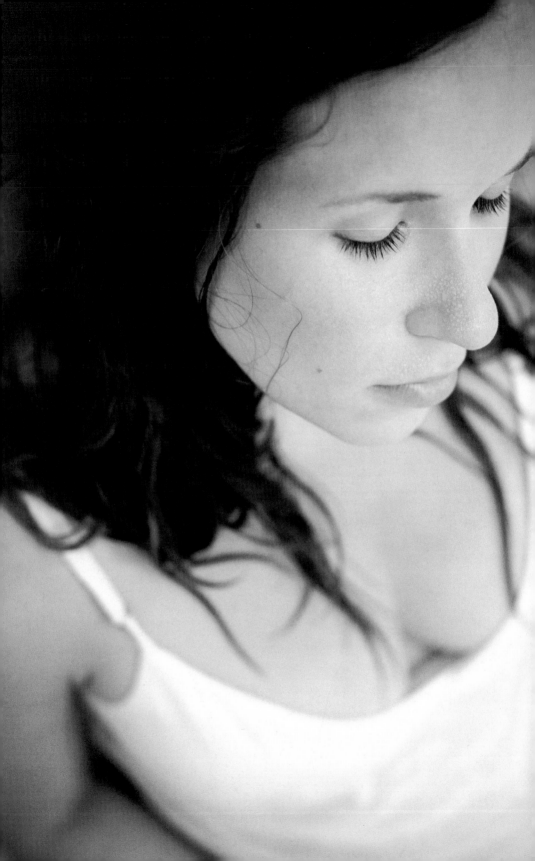

Surrender

*close your eyes
and bring your focus within*

YOUR BODY ༄

At this stage, you may experience a number of things to let you know things are going to be getting started. Firstly, you may be having more and more Braxton Hicks contractions. Don't be fooled into thinking these aren't real. Every contraction you have does something. They are real, even the ones you have had earlier in the pregnancy, but not all lead to the birth that day. At this stage of the game however, your contractions are all coming with the intention of getting your baby out of your body. They are a way of acclimating your body to the sensations and feeling of the surges to come that will gradually get stronger and longer.

Secondly, you may experience something called a "bloody show," where the mucus plug comes out and you have slight bleeding. Although this is a good sign of things coming, this does not mean you are in labor.

Thirdly, your water may break. How do you know if your water has broken? You will feel a gush of water literally run down your leg. It's a lot of water usually, so it's hard to mistake it for anything else. If your water breaks, call your midwife or check in with your doctor and birthing support team.

Contractions, or what I will call surges (which I learned from my hypbirth sessions), are a very distinctive feeling. Your lower abdomen tightens up and gets very hard and then it goes away. At first, these may not stop you in your tracks, and may just be something you notice. Usually in the beginning of early labor, you will be able to carry on with your daily activities (and should, because this could go on for hours). Once you have a regular rhythm to your surges, where they are coming every ten minutes or so, start bringing your focus to the pending birth. You may want to start laboring in a warm tub of water or on a birthing ball, but use the in-between time to make sure you have all you need and that your birthing team is in place to support you in every way.

YOUR BABY ⌒

At the end of this week, your baby is pretty well-cooked and can join the world really any time. According to Dr. Biter and many other experts, thirty-seven weeks is considered full term. So if you have your baby anytime between thirty-seven and forty-two weeks, you are fine and your baby is developed enough to enter the world and be healthy. These last weeks are really spent packing on pounds, so anywhere in this range is good.

YOUR SPIRIT ⌒

There are five stages of labor: (1) early, (2) active, (3) transition that includes pushing the baby out, (4) delivery of the placenta, and (5) recovery. (See the stages of labor on page 327 for more detail.) Each of these phases requires a level of surrender. Once you realize you are in labor and surges (also known as contractions) are coming, it's game time. This is when everything else in the world is put aside and all that matters is birthing your baby. We have done a lot of work throughout the book on preparing for this big day. When it finally arrives, you should be ready to put on that empowerment necklace and do the work that needs to be done.

WEEK 37 ⌒

Here we go. Once your early labor crosses that bridge to where you are no longer chit-chatting, organizing, cleaning, or setting stuff up, you are settling into the process and ready to do that deep surrender. What does that mean? Well, it means that you are now in a place of complete trust and willingness to let your power win over fear, your strength conquer your weaknesses. When you close your eyes, find that safe place from your visualization, a place that comforts you, listen to some type of music that inspires you. I always had only one song (different for each child) playing at the births and this song became "our song."

Reflections

When we are afraid of something, our bodies usually tense up, rather than go limp. When we go limp, we are in a trusting space, where we can feel vulnerable and loose. This is where you need to surrender to. The loose place, not the tense, fearful place. Now, this may go against your instincts because of every message you have ever gotten about birth being a scary and painful thing. There is such thing as a painless birth, Mama, if you believe, trust and ride each surge as a wave totally breathing into them and pushing down, rather than tensing up. I have had a painless birth, so I know it can happen. I have also had painful births. When I birthed my third child, Bodhi, I was determined to try this concept of painless birth.

The word pain-less, doesn't mean no pain at all, it means less pain than normal. I went into it trusting, doing my meditations, being focused and determined to surrender to the process. The entire birth lasted two hours, start to finish, with about ten major surges, where I literally melted into each one. I did not resist, even though my mind was telling me to. I resisted those thoughts and surrendered to my body. After these ten surges or so, I felt the urge to push, and gave three hard pushes, and out he flew. The entire experience was quick, easy and full of intention. I willed that to happen, and my husband supported me in this process and was there to champion me through it. He was my constant reminder—looking into his eyes, hearing him say I could do it and reminding me to surrender into each surge, was what led me through the birthing tunnel with such ease.

So let's recap ... **SURRENDER!** Do not resist ... literally push into the surge, rather than pull away from it! You can do it, Mama! Use your voice and your breath awareness to keep you centered and focused.

Ideas

· If you are having a home birth, make sure your big tub of supplies is in the birthing space so your midwife can have easy access to everything she needs. (Oh, just an FYI, the midwives clean everything up! I get asked that question so much ... who cleans up all the mess? It's surprisingly a pretty contained mess, but either way, they do it!)

- Set up a small birthing altar with the most important symbols of strength and power on it that will serve as a touchstone or focal point during labor. Light a couple of candles to remind you of your will and determination.

- Get your phone tree buzzing with the news that things are getting started and ask those who can to bathe in the salts of your blessing-way and light candles sending you powerful birthing energy. Your sister circle gathering to support you will help you! Let them help, either from afar or at the actual birth. Whatever you have decided to do, just allow them to be your support.

journal on

Surrender

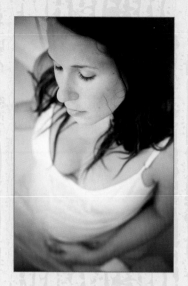

What does it mean to you to completely surrender to your body and trust the universe?

close your eyes and bring your focus within

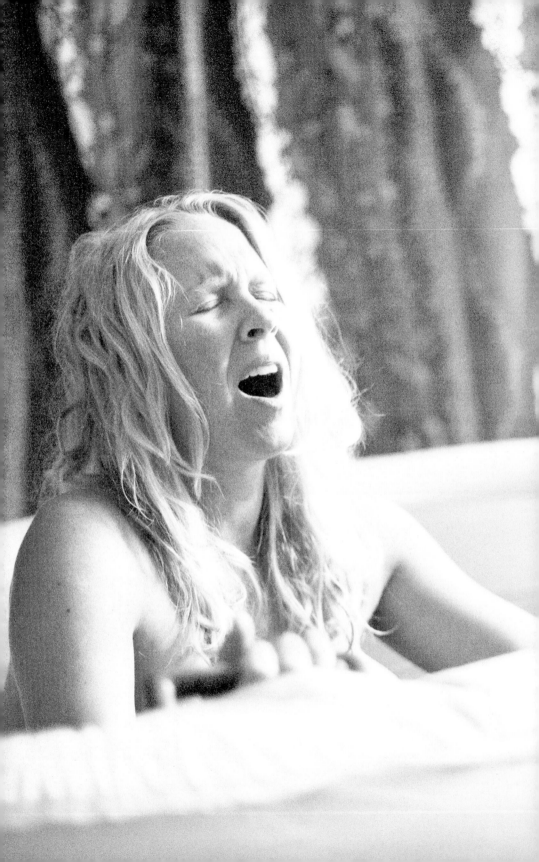

Surges

*ride the waves and let your body
do the work it's meant to do*

YOUR BODY ❧

You are now in active labor—every surge does something and has a purpose. These surges are thinning your cervix or doing what is called "effacing." Know that women have been birthing babies for centuries, and they all belong to a sacred tribe that you will be entering now. The medical community often strips women of their power to be able to birth naturally, but your body holds ancient wisdom within your womb and it knows *exactly* what to do. You can have a painless, beautiful birth, if that is your will. Your surges are likely three to five minutes apart now and are lasting about sixty seconds. These are intense surges, but manageable. Take each one completed as an accomplishment and know that the end result of these is pushing out your baby.

Did you know? At a home birth or birth-center birth, you can labor any way you like, whether it's in the tub, the shower, on a birthing ball, walking, sitting, or lying down. You are encouraged to do whatever you need to do. Some hospitals are also now progressing to understand that laboring women may need to be in several different positions to labor and will encourage them to try different positions. Also, consider gravity. The baby needs to be pushed out, so lying on your back in a bed is often not the best or most comfortable way to birth. Standing, squatting, or birthing in the water tend to be more effective birthing positions.

YOUR BABY ❧

Your baby is in full working mode during active labor, as she is moving her way down the birth canal helping you to push her little being into the world. There is going to be intense feelings when this is happening, both physically and mentally. It's an exhausting process, and a laboring mother needs to make sure she rests in between surges.

YOUR SPIRIT ❧

You will know when you are in active labor because nothing else matters to you except your labor. You are now face to face with everything you practiced and learned throughout the pregnancy and are being called upon by the universe to trust, surrender, and birth your baby. This is the time to pull out that tool bag and use everything you've got. The breathing techniques, the meditations, the visualization work, the mantras, and the calling in of sisters past who have birthed before you. All of these are your tools and yours alone to use as you wish. There is no shame in any type of birth and, although natural birth is best for you and baby, that is not always possible. Be in the moment and be present with your birth and do what you need to do, plain and simple.

WEEK 38

You are standing at the crossroads right now and can either go down the road of powerful woman or fearful woman. Which path will you choose? It is not easy to choose going through the fire, but when you do, you will not believe that feeling you have after birthing your baby. It is amazing and empowering and really takes you to a new level of woman. This goes for all women who birth a baby, no matter how you birth them, in a hospital, at home, in a birthing center, swimming with dolphins, on a beach, in a car, or through a C-section. What-ever your circumstances are, you are entering the tribe of women who have given birth and that alone gets you in the club, and gives you a one-way ticket to the journey of motherhood. Welcome, as you are the guest of honor tonight, and as we all raise our glasses to you in rever-ence and awe, let me just say that we are all very proud of you.

Reflections

If you have done the emotional work of preparing for this baby and feel ready to give birth, you will have a far easier time than if you come to the table unprepared. It's like taking a test you have not stud-ied for—you may get some of the answers, but not feel good about the experience and will likely feel like your are "winging" it. The point of this book is to help you feel prepared emotionally, spiritually, and physically to birth your baby and enter motherhood. Just because I suggest that birth can be pain-*less,* does not mean it's not the hardest work you will ever do, because it is. That is why it is so important that with each surge you ride through, have a little mini-celebration in your head because that means you are doing it, sister! Even in your darkest moments when you thought you could never do this in a million years, you are doing it! Here and now.

Ideas

• Remember that each surge moves you closer to meeting your baby. Have your partner tell you when each surge is starting and ending. This will help you gauge each one.

• Try to stay away from updates—meaning try not to ask your practitioner to keep "checking" you to see how far along you are. That is a mind game that can have weird results. The truth is that there is no way to really tell how long it will take, so don't worry about it—just move through each one and prepare your body for pushing.

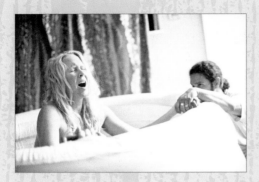

journal on

Surges

Can you ride the waves of
these surges? What are your
fears around this process?

ride the waves and let your body do the work it's meant to do _journal on_

Surges

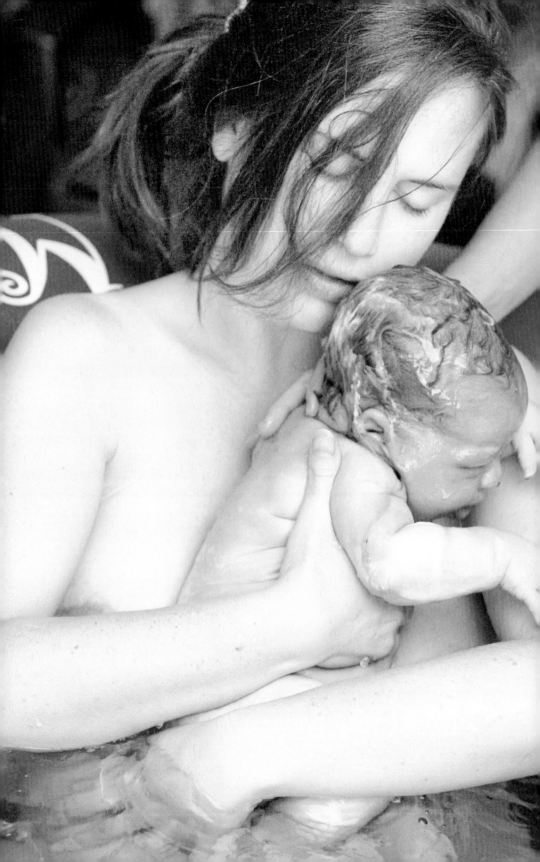

Birth

*call upon your inner strength
to get the job done*

YOUR BODY ～

Your body has moved through every single phase of this experience and is now ready to complete the cycle. You have been having surges for a while and are likely moving into the transition phase as you hit eight to ten centimeters dilated and are almost entirely effaced. You will have longer surges, about sixty to ninety seconds each, and they will come about every two minutes.

BIRTH EUPHORIA: TIPS ON ENJOYING YOUR LABOR AND DELIVERY

BY CHRISTY FUNK

During birth

- Completely surrender to the process.

- Make sure that your body is limp and loose, and that you are not storing tension anywhere in the body.

- Invite only those who are in alignment with your birth wishes to your birth.

- Keep things simple. The most important thing you can do is to tune into that deep place in your mind and concentrate on your breath and communicating with baby.

- Focus on your breath and do not allow fear to alter your breathwork. If you can control and monitor your breath and continue to focus on it, your body will relax enough to deliver your baby without complications.

- Let your baby know that you are there for her and that the world is a safe place to come out.

- Roll with the contractions and think of them as surges, rather than pain. Try to visualize them as waves and ride them instead of fighting them. The more you can relax your body, the easier the pathway for delivery is. If you focus on the pain, then more pain will come. Push into the surge opening your body, rather than contracting during the surge, which will slow everything down.

- Enjoy the process and make it playful. Feel every part of your body and marvel at how it is all working together to bring your baby closer to you.

YOUR BABY ❧

The baby is working just as hard as you are to move through the birth canal to meet you. This is not a one-person show and your baby is seriously working hard to help you and to get on out of there and into the world. During this phase, when you begin to crown, you may feel perineal burning sensations. When you feel that, it's a good sign that your baby is almost here. Push past the burning. Remember that when you are in labor, push past the burning feeling and very soon after that your baby will slide into the world.

YOUR SPIRIT ❧

This is it ... transition and pushing your baby into the world. How will you face this challenge? What will you do to move past your fear and do the woman's work that is required for your baby to be in your arms? Remember that when you are in this transition phase, it means your baby is *very* near and although you may be hitting that place of exhaustion and feeling overwhelmed, this is the time to dig deep and bring out your warrior goddess and get the job done. Yell, roar, laugh, play, be silent, moan, whatever it takes to do *your* work. Try to maintain short breaths so you maintain the oxygen going to your brain and don't get lightheaded. A great technique I learned from hypbirth is that every time I had a "surge," my husband would look at me and remind me to breathe *into* the surge, and not to pull away from it. This helped as a constant reminder to stay in the present moment with my surges and roll with them, like riding a wave.

WEEK 39 ⊙〜

As you enter this last phase of labor just remember all that you have worked toward and that you are all-powerful and your body is made to do this work. Your body has the knowledge of birthing imprinted into your bones and all you have to do is show up and trust! After your baby has come into the world, you will also deliver the placenta. You will have contractions and then deliver it.

Reflections

One of the most beautiful things about being in labor and especially about the transition stage, is that for these moments you are 100 percent present. You know everything your body is doing and you are more aware than ever about what is happening in that exact moment. You are alive with fierce energy and are communing with all elements and the divine feminine. That is actually pure magic. Honor this sacred experience.

BEING BORN IS IMPORTANT *by Carl Sandberg*

Being born is important
You who have stood at the bedposts
and seen a mother on her high harvest day,
the day of the most golden of harvest moons for her.
You who have seen the new wet child
dried behind the ears,
swaddled in soft fresh garments,
pursing its lips and sending a groping mouth
toward nipples where white milk is ready.
You who have seen this love's payday
of wild toiling and sweet agonizing.
You know being born is important.
You know that nothing else was ever so important to you.
You understand that the payday of love is so old,
So involved, so traced with circles of the moon,
So cunning with the secrets of the salts of the blood.
It must be older than the moon, older than salt.

Ideas

· Placenta pills: You can have your placenta dried out and encapsulated into pills. This will assist in your recovery and boost your energy. Even if you deliver in the hospital, you can ask them to save your placenta.

· You may want to ask a friend or a photographer to come to the birth to photograph your baby coming into the world.

· Ask someone from your birthing support team to make sure there is a nice, warm, healthy soup waiting for you for after giving birth. A vegetable broth soup with kale would be great to pack in a little extra iron boost.

T-Shirt Pairing

Sacred Pregnancy Tees by Erin Wallace at Tiny Twist Creative
www.tinytwist.com or
www.sacredpregancy.com

A portion of the sales of these organic tees goes to supporting a woman's ability to birth the way she wants to.

journal on

Your Birth Story

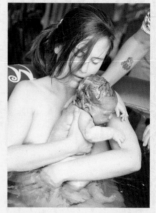

You did it! Plain and simple, your body held the knowledge to help you create a new little life, and YOU stepped into your full womanhood, pulled from your deepest self and birthed your baby. Welcome to the tribe. Please use this section to tell your birth story. Take a few quiet moments to document your journey through the last hours of your pregnancy and what you remember about the birth itself and how you felt those first moments you held your little baby. This process is important for your transition out of pregnancy and into motherhood. It will allow you a treasured keepsake for years to come. Some questions that may help you get started are:

1. What time did you go into labor and how did you know you were in labor?

2. What did the surges feel like and who was there supporting you?

3. What was the setting like where you were laboring?

4. How did you manage the surges?

5. How long were you in labor?

6. What were the thoughts going through your head during the laboring process? Did you feel empowered during the process?

7. How long did you push before your baby came out?

8. Were there any complications?

9. What time was your baby born and how much did your baby weigh?

call upon your inner strength to get the job done

journal on

Your Birth Story

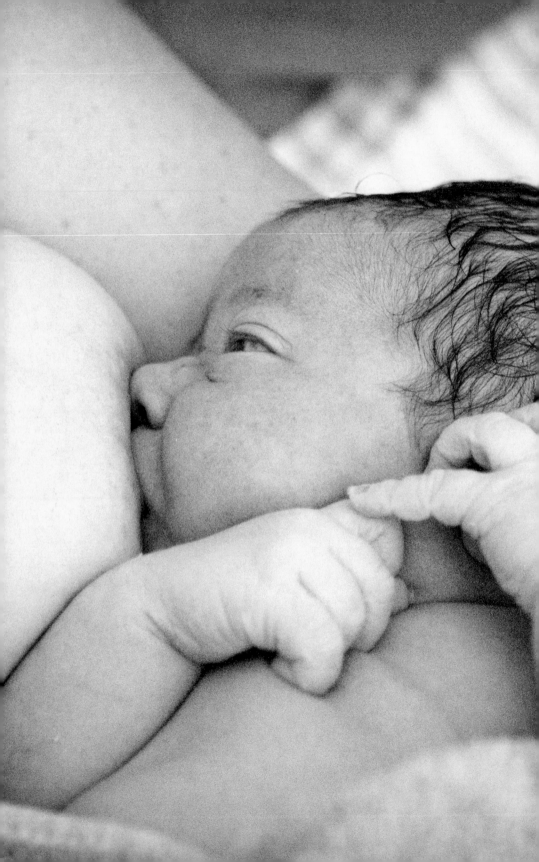

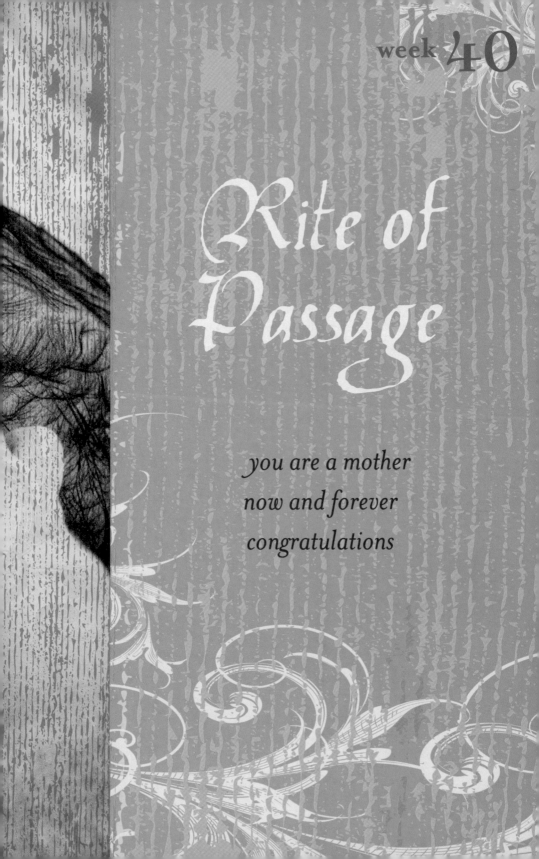

Rite of Passage

you are a mother

now and forever

congratulations

YOUR BODY ℰ⌒⌐

So you have birthed your baby and now you hold your little sweetie in your arms, and are likely overwhelmed with joy and exhaustion. Your body has just worked harder than it probably ever has or ever will and needs some recovery time. If you decide to have your placenta turned into pills, this will help in your recovery and healing. What your body needs is sleep, good food, and comfort. It is normal for you to be pretty sore, and a great healing thing to do after a birth is to soak in a sitz bath, which is basically a warm bath with herb-infused water. See Resources on page 321 to learn where to get them. Also, have a peri-bottle next to the toilet to use instead of wiping. This is a little water bottle that you can use to squirt yourself clean. Warm water in these bottles works best. Also have large sanitary pads available for use. You will likely bleed heavily for a few days and then at the end of the first week, the bleeding will taper way down. It's wise to keep sheets or towels under you on your bed during those first few days.

YOUR BABY ℰ⌒⌐

Your baby is already hungry! Your breastmilk does not actually come in for a couple of days after the baby is born, and those first few days the baby is drinking what is called *colostrum,* which is filled with antibodies that help build her immune system. Your body produces the perfect food for your baby. Isn't that incredible? There is no other time in your child's life when they will get better nutrition that right now. Breastmilk is the superfood your baby needs. Breast-feeding also helps your uterus go back into place and helps you lose weight naturally. Your baby will sleep a lot during these first few weeks and gradually will awaken to the world around her. She will regulate her body clock with yours if you allow that to just happen naturally. Co-sleeping helps this out tremendously. Your baby will likely sleep when you do if you co-sleep. Keep your house calm and peaceful, but not too quiet. Keep conversations going in the same room that your baby is sleeping in so they are used to a little noise when they doze off. If you have other children, you have a built-in noise factor to consider, but honestly babies and kids adapt to their environment, and as long as it's a loving and peaceful space, the world is right and they are happy.

YOUR SPIRIT ⌒◡

Be proud of yourself and what you just did. It is an amazing task that you conquered. You brought a new life into the world. These first few weeks can be emotional ones as your hormones are still out of whack, so make sure to recognize your emotions may be slightly off-kilter. Keep taking your prenatal New Chapter vitamins and the placenta pills, which will really help regulate you.

WEEK 40 ⌒◡

You are finally holding your little baby, and that is a miracle and a huge accomplishment. In almost every culture, giving birth is seen as a rite of passage, a journey from maiden to mother. You now live in the mother-world and are no longer living in the realm of maiden, so embrace your new social standing with the awe and reverence it deserves. Hopefully you have worked out the details of sleeping, changing diapers, and breast-feeding, so now you can settle into the new life together that will soon become routine. Having four children, I have seen how fast the time goes and am so grateful I spent as much time as I could holding my babies, sleeping with them just cuddled right up in my arms all night. Those days are quickly ending, and I know it is something I will deeply miss. Enjoy every moment of breast-feeding, holding and rocking your baby to sleep, and all the in between times when she is just down right adorable.

Reflections

Now that baby is here, consider having a small hibernation fest. The two of you just met and although so many people want to come and meet the baby, try to keep everyone at bay for a little while. This will allow the two of you to bond and connect without outside distractions. Your partner is also just meeting the baby and needs alone, quiet time to bond with the baby. After my last baby, River, was born, my midwife wrapped him in a blanket and a diaper and we did not even put clothes on him for two days. I remember just holding him snuggled up next to me in that soft, little blanket. Not much has changed, as he still snuggles up for his mommy milk seventeen months later, but those few days are just so intensely magical and I would encourage you to inhale those moments with every ounce of energy you have. My husband and I spent one whole day just staring at our daughter Lotus after she was born. We sat on the couch, taking turns holding her and just marveled at her. It was a day I will never forget.

Ideas

- You may want to consider wrapping your belly with a postpartum wrap. In many cultures, for the first six weeks after a woman gives birth, her belly is wrapped tightly with a long piece of fabric to help her belly go back into shape and to support her healing. Try the Moby Belly Postpartum Wrap for a beautiful wrap that you can show off to the world, letting them know you just had a baby.

- Get the food tree going. Hopefully one of your sisters from your birthing support team will arrange this with your community of friends. Having folks drop off prepared meals is one of the greatest gifts you can give new parents. Cooking and cleaning get moved to the back burner during those first few weeks, so whatever help you can get in that area is well worth it.

Music Pairing

Best lullaby CDs

It's A Big World by Renee and Jeremy (so sweet!)

Lullabies by Jewell

Rite of Passage

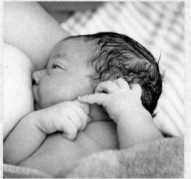

Now that you are holding your baby in your arms, how do you want to welcome her or him to the world? Take a moment to write down who were the first visitors and what those first moments of your meeting was like for you.

you are a mother now and forever

congratulations

Journal on
Rite of Passage

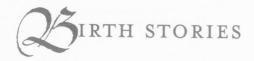# BIRTH STORIES

BIRTH OF RUMI ℮⁓

TOLD BY HIS MOTHER, CHRISTY FUNK

Within moments I felt a rush through my abdomen. My eyes snapped out of the daze of floating in the water for about an hour, bathing in ecstasy, my body weightless in a sea of warmth. I exclaimed, "The baby is coming! The baby is coming! I am not pushing. Baby is coming!" I remember the heat as my baby descended into the birth canal, caressing my body, widening his passageway and preparing for his arrival. I was startled out of my blissful state and remember thinking that I had only read about this experience in natural childbirth books and here my body was re-creating what others universally have felt before. I closed my eyes positioned my hands and chanted a Kundalini chant: God and Me, Me and God are one. My baby had spoken to me and told me to get ready. He was ready to meet his co-creators.

The day before my delivery, I woke up to call my midwife. Enough, I told her as I nursed my toddler, we need to get this moving. I have had enough. She sent me off to the local health food store to pickup some herbal tinctures to jumpstart the process. I took them before lunch and then settled down for a nap with my son. I began to feel some subtle sensations, but nothing worth calling her about. My large belly was uncomfortable and after a pregnancy riddled with back pain, I was ready to get my little baby out.

Later that day I was breathing, squatting, talking on the phone and making something to eat in the kitchen. My friend in New York had the pleasure of hearing me suddenly take a deep breath and then con-

tinue my conversation. After that conversation ended I called up
another friend. We had a lot of catching up to do and for whatever
reason, I was not making the connection that perhaps I was in labor.
After dinner I was laying on my bed to get a massage from a friend
while Juan read to my son in the other room. Five minutes, four minutes, two minutes apart, Nicki called out to my husband. He showed
up at the doorway looking at me curled and relaxed on the bed, drinking in the luxury of a sweet massage. Can we call Sue (our midwife)
now, he asks me. Well O.K., I tell him, still certain there was nothing really going on with me. Within a half an hour Sue and her daughter are at my home. The contractions stopped. Cold turkey. I was pre-
scribed a small glass of wine, a bath and instructions to go to bed. I
obliged, my swollen belly pressing against my husband as he cradled
my son. We were all asleep by 10 p.m.

My arm was lightly draped across my husbands waist. Deep breath,
snippet of sleep, deep breath, snippet of sleep. I was actually sleeping between contractions. Wild. I had heard about this and thought
it was impossible, yet here I was sleeping through waves of contractions. At one point I got up to go to the bathroom. Whew, I mumbled
to myself, this is intense. Maybe I shouldn't have anymore kids. This is
strong. Off I went to pee, came back to bed and just took many more
deep breaths without waking my husband, without screaming, moan-
ing or asking for help. In the middle of that dark night it was me, my
breath and my little baby inhaling and exhaling the beauty of labor.
I was in that deep place in my soul, trusting my body and in those
moments I was fully present. There was no fear of what was to come

and no drama about the jabs of intensity heating my womb. I was there with my child enveloped in that mysterious place where women have come before me, embracing birth with sheer surrender and joy. Magical.

Then it happened. At 3:30 a.m. my water gushed out drenching the bed. Woosh! Juan, I called out, my water! I got onto all fours, he checked to see if my cord was O.K. and then started to get the pool ready. My son woke up and was lying on the bed staring at me. Deep breath in, Mommy is having a baby I told him smiling, deep breath out. His angelic face looked at me puzzled but not scared. Fear wasn't anywhere near this home. By 4 a.m. Sue and her daughter arrived. Soon after Sue's assistant, Katie, showed up. I began to show signs of, well, euphoria.

It started with Sue. I started singing. Not ballads or anything remotely romantic. Real songs like "Wheels on the Bus" and classic 1970s rock songs. Anything that would pop into my little laboring mind would then be thrust forward with my vocal cords. The entire birth team would receive their personalized versions of my improvisations. It felt good to be vocal, to be funny, to make this experience light and joyful. So I sang. However, I wasn't dancing. I was laying on my side while Sue massaged my back and in between my singing would soothingly talk to me. Yes just ride the wave Christy. Here comes another one, just ride it. Now you are going down. Gentle and encouraging she never left my side. When I had to go to the bathroom, my body instantly weighing a ton, I grabbed on to her and asked her to be my mother. She smiled and hugged me.

The kiddie pool was ready and they helped me in. I sank into the water and instantly my songbird career stopped. It was as if someone had dipped me in heaven. My body relaxed with no effort, meshing with the perfection of the water. Was I dreaming or could anything be so divine as to make me feel utterly delicious? My euphoria was allowing me to close my eyes, smile and breathe deeper into my soul. My friend who showed up, her back resting on the wall next to the pool, thought my labor stalled. I was so quiet. Time rolled with a subtle motion. Finally Sue instructed my husband to get into the water.

I needed some support to hold me up as my arm was getting tired. Then things really started to move.

My silence was broken with deep, powerful, and bellowing animal sounds. So strong that at one point my son, propped next to the pool, almost got frightened. That's when Sue told him that Mommy was pretending to be a lion. The birth team chimed in with their own lion sounds and my son smiled and continued to watch me. I was getting closer. I could feel it. My baby was coming.

He slid out into the water, slipping straight into my arms. I would later find out that the cord was wrapped around his neck twice, but Sue had quickly un-wrapped it. I now had my beautiful baby boy in my arms. He looks like a Cuban boxer, I exclaimed to everyone. Sue looked at him and mumbled something about him being big. Juan and I just smiled and cooed at this little boy with his cowlick and rounded face, lapping in the gushes of universal love. Our son was born at home. He was safe. We were in love.

After the big meal my mother prepared for my family and birth team, I nestled in bed with Rumi still elated from the whole experience. I had birthed a 10-pound, 12-ounce baby at home in the water! My midwife left after several hours and I knew she was taking home with her a birth story that she would never forget. I remember her telling us, after Rumi was born, that we were not alone in that room. That without a doubt there was something much bigger than ourselves who had come to bless us with nothing short of a miracle. I would have been a C-section plain and simple, had I gone through standard hospital practice. I would have been classified as high-risk and a scheduled C-section would have erased my personal birth plan for what the medical world would have proclaimed as impossible. But there we were, baby and I perfectly healthy and happy after about five hours of active labor. My body knew what to do, my baby knew how to be birthed and there is not a soul on this earth who could negate that. No emergency C-section, no drama, just a baby slipping into the world with love and acceptance.

There is something quite phenomenal when a woman delivers her baby without intervention. It is almost impossible to put into words because the deep rooted feelings are so profound, almost primitive in nature, that books, poems and the written word have tried to capture that instant-of-a-moment when our babies come into the world naturally. A woman who chooses to have a baby naturally is proclaiming that she is in alignment with her body and soul and that her body is a sheer force of ability to do what women have done since the beginning of time. We grab that power and engulf its essence to be able to surrender to the innate knowledge we all have. Once we acknowledge that our bodies were designed to deliver, we can accept it and then move on to surrender. We are vehicles of which babies come into the world, so we need to let them navigate through that birth canal with an open license. When we birth in this realm, the gift is beyond euphoric. Universally it gathers us as women sharing a common thread and this powerful force is what makes the earth shift every moment a baby is born. Every little moment.

BIRTH OF ROMEO ℮◡◞

TOLD BY HIS MOTHER TNAH LOUISE

My birthing journey began in my third month of pregnancy when I moved to a remote village on the Pacific side of Costa Rica named Montezuma. I had fantasized about having my baby natural in a beautiful fresh water spring among all the creatures of the land, only to have been shot down by the reality of the potential harm due to bacteria lurking in the water.

During my fifth month I had to endure a brutal emergency trip to the hospital, which ended up being a five hour journey by bumpy dirt roads and a scheduled ferry to cross the Nicoya. My arrival to the hospital was so bleak, I knew I had to plan for a very different birth experience because there would be no way I would give birth in such an oppressive place. I was told early on by the doctor who gave me my final ultra sound that our baby was likely to be born without fingers on his right hand. Naturally this saddened our heart, especially his father who longed to teach his child guitar. Never the less I stayed centered and visualized a happy healthy baby throughout my entire pregnancy.

My search to find a midwife in my small village was unsuccessful, but I found an American nurse and an American mother who had ten children on the same private stretch of beach all on her own about an hour's journey away. They were very excited to open up their Swiss Family Robinson house to us and deliver our child. To think that the cost for this amazing birthing experience was going to be a mere $250.00, wow! I snorkeled and swam at least three to four hours a day religiously, it was the only relief I found, floating in the water and practicing my breathing techniques under water with my snorkeling gear, so physically I was fit for the experience. Music and dance was a must, I remained very active.

As my due date came and went I naturally became impatient because I had none of the signs that indicated going into labor. On the morning of March 15, 1995, I woke up full of energy, not only was nesting in full effect, I decided to stay out late that night at our restaurant Muy Nice for a weekly event called Cafe Mambo with live music. I almost continued my night with dancing at the local disco but decided to return home instead arriving around midnight. Not having all the books around to educate myself I thought I had peed my pants, only to find that my water bag had broke and I had begun my first phase of labor.

The late painter Luciana Martinez Della Rosa who had traveled from NYC to accompany me and document the birth was picked up off the dance floor of the disco and off we drove an hour on the bumpy dirt roads guided only by the brightness of the moon. We arrived at our destination at around 2:30 a.m. only to find that another mother had also gone into labor and the room they had prepared for me was in use. All I wanted to do was walk, and walk some more. Naked, I walked along the private beach's coast line and watched the sun rise with Tony and Luciana, and continued to walk up and down 200 stairs back and forth to combat my pain! When it came down to the hardest part of labor I could no longer make it back up the stairs and preparations for a beach delivery had to be made.

Not having slept a wink, and using up most of my energy walking, I was completely delirious as I tried to ride the waves of pain. My eyes were rolled in the back of my head, as I howled like the howler monkeys up high in the trees, deep and tribal like from the most primal part of my being. I recall trying to sleep through the eternal 30 seconds of the final pushing. Within a half hour of six strong pushes I gave birth, squatting, to a healthy baby boy. In that moment tears flowed down my face as I laid eyes on Romeo as he was caught by his father. After downing a half bottle of honey and two gallons of apple juice my hard work had paid off, at 11:36 a.m. Romeo came out looking absolutely beautiful! Not wrinkled like most newborns, eyes wide open, and all ten fingers intact. I did it! I gave birth naturally, to a 8-pound, 4-ounce bountiful baby boy named Romeo on a sprawling beach in Pochotte, Costa Rica. Born under a full moon along with three other babies, a colt, and one litter of kittens. It is said that a full moon's gravitational pull is known to activate labor in both humans and animals, so true indeed!

My joy was somewhat interrupted as I was given two pitocin shots to help tighten my uterus which did not seem to work as I lost too much blood. We had to work fast, getting a helicopter in the middle of nowhere was not an option! When there are no options it is amazing what we are capable of, my midwives were professionals and single handedly, literally, massaged my uterus closed. Funny to think that Romeo, who is nearing seventeen now, has been blessed with a the gift of playing the violin, viola, mandolin, and guitar. I believe it was our faith and determination to Source that made this possible! Romeo is the oldest of four brothers, the other three Domenico, Paolo, and Nicolai were all water births in the comfort of our home and all were beautiful and unique birthing experiences that I will forever cherish.

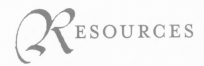

RESOURCES

PREGNANCY ❧

Sacred Pregnancy Website
www.sacredpregnancy.com

Conscious Conception and Pregnancy
consciousconceptionandpregnancy.com/index.html

Conscious Pre-Conception, Pregnancy and Birth
www.wondersofthewomb.com

American College of Nurse Midwives
www.acnm.org

BiniBirth
binibirth.com

New Chapter Prenatal Vitamins
newchapter.com/prenatal

Nordic Naturals Prental DHA Vitamins
Nordic Naturals Pregnancy Omega-3 Vitamins
www.nordicnaturals.com

Preganancy Awareness Month
www.preganancyawareness.com

The Sanctuary Birth and Family Wellness Center—they can also do
placenta pills
birthsanctuary.com

Natural Childbirth
www.naturalchildbirth.org

Water Birth International
www.waterbirth.org

Home Birth Videos
www.homebirthvideos.com

The Business of Being Born documentary, by Ricki Lake and Abby Epstein
thebusinessofbeingborn.com

Birthing Ball
doulashop.com

Home Birth Kit
homebirthkits.com

Birthing From Within
birthingfromwithin.com

Justine Serebrin: Los Angeles based artist and painter of pregnant mama's bellys.
www.justineserebrin.com

Alisa Starkweather's Red Tent Movement
alisastarkweather.comOpen-Hearted Music and Information for Pregnancy and Birth
www.baby-welcoming.com

Joanne Ameya Cohen- Teacher, Herbalist, Flower Essence Practitioner and Birth Doula. Also, Encapsulates Placentas for Post-Partum Health
www.sacredpassageways.com

Birth Balance
birthbalance.com/home.asp

Dr. Biter Birth Center / San Diego
babiesbytheseaboutique.com

The Sacred Garden, Maui. The Sacred Garden on Maui is a healing sanctuary operated by the Divine Nature Alliance, a public charity non-profit.
www.SacredGardenMaui.com

mom, BABY, AND pARENTING ⌒

Green Nest and Healthy Home advocate
www.greenhugs.net

Attachment Parenting International
attachmentparenting.org/

Comprehensive Resource for Healthy Living and Detoxifying
Your Environment

www.healthychild.org

Holistic Moms Network
holisticmoms.org

La Leche League
www.lalecheleague.org

Earth Mama Angel baby
earthmamaangelbaby.com/pregnancy

Belly Sprout
bellysprout.com

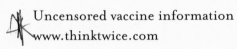

Uncensored vaccine information
www.thinktwice.com

Cloth diapers / Sloomb
sloomb.com

GDiapers
www.gdiapers.com

Nature Baby Clothes
naturebaby.com/us/

Innovative Baby
www.innovativebaby.com

Nova Natural Toys
novanatural.com

Episencials
episencial.com

Moby Wraps for baby and postpartum by Moby and Anni Daulter
mobywrap.com

Kelly Wells Cloth Diapering Expert
kellywels.com

Eco Nuts
econutssoap.com

EcoBaby Planning and Concierge with Melanie Monroe
www.ecobabyplanning.com

Happy Dough Lucky (Email owner Rheiana Lenox Alderette and tell her I sent you, and that you are pregnant and need a great doughnut sent your way!)
www.facebook.com/happydoughlucky

Motherhood, the Musical
www.motherhoodthemusical.com

Sunday Set Up
with Kathy Kaehler

PHOTOGRAPHERS ❧

Elena Rego (primary)
www.elenarego.com

Alexandra DeFurio (primary)
www.defuriophotography.com

Cristy Nielsen (contributor)
www.nielsensonline.com

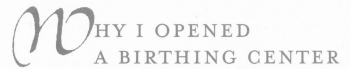

WHY I OPENED A BIRTHING CENTER

Dr. Robert Biter, MD

"Dr. Robert Biter Stands for Women"

This was on a picket sign outside the hospital where I was fired for standing up for women's rights to birth babies how they want!

The decision to build a birthing center was an evolutionary one. Throughout my career, I have been tutored by the amazing women and their partners who have been transformed by their births, who have fought for respect and safety in their birthing experiences and who live their lives differently as parents because of the experience in becoming parents. I have learned that hospitals are not inherently programmed to honor birth or death, the two most amazingly human experiences that we all have and will experience. I know that we can do better. Babies by the Sea Birthing Center will hopefully continue the sea of change that has begun years before I ever was accepted into medical school or delivered my first baby. I hope to advance the works of Mardsen Wagner and Ina May Gaskin and all those amazing families who first taught me that birth is the greatest opportunity for all of us to begin life anew. While I support and offer home births in my practice, I also realize that more families can be helped in a birthing center that consolidates our resources. I hope to set an example for other like-minded doctors and midwives who want to make a difference in how women are treated in pregnancy and childbirth and are able to rebuild a new system rooted in truth and love, rather than fear and manipulation. We will protect normal at Babies by the Sea Birthing Center and recognize when an abnormal process or pathology exists, which rarely does, and transfer to a hospital only when needed.

C-Section Rate Debate

DR. ROBERT BITER, MD

The rising rates of Cesarean deliveries exactly mirrors the increasing reliance upon technology and inductions. What remains interesting is that despite the belief that interventions are powerful tools to somehow protect a woman or her baby from a normal process, these interventions have only increased exposure to major surgery and have done nothing to improve our maternal or neonatal outcomes. To imagine that the United States cannot provide better pregnancy care than many developing countries points exactly to the hospital based physicians' unwillingness to consider than nature is more powerful than humankind. It would be interesting to witness what would happen to Cesarean rates and maternal neonatal outcomes if doctors and hospitals were subjected to real peer review, where only indicated surgical procedures could be performed just as any other medical surgical specialty.

I support the standard of care that pregnancy is considered full term from 37 weeks until 42 weeks gestation. I find it concerning that providers choose to follow literature based guidelines only when convenient to their schedules or plan of care. Intervention of any type should be carefully chosen and should only occur when indicated and after a full informed discussion of the risks and benefits takes place.

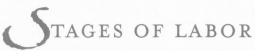

STAGES OF LABOR

Aleksandra Evanguelidi LM, CPM

Clinical Director, The Sanctuary Birth and Family Wellness Center

LABOR OF LOVE

Or maybe more like the labor of a lifetime. Either way, the result is indeed the love of a lifetime, and for that, we give it everything we've got. There are no "you can expect it to go this way" conversations that hold up any salt when it comes to describing this awesome experience since every woman will birth uniquely each time she steps up to bat. So, with that as my caveat, I am going to try and describe the stages of labor as best I can.

EARLY LABOR

This is when you think you might be warming up. You might be experiencing your bowels evacuating, lots of Braxton Hicks contractions, possibly some uterine cramps that are low, reminding you of those you would have around your menses. My best piece of advice: GO TO SLEEP. The most common reaction to this exciting change in action is to get the watch out and start the timing process. BAD IDEA. Early labor can go on for days, sometimes weeks. This might be the number one reason why women get epidurals for pain relief—it's not that they can't handle the pain of labor; it's that they are so tired by the time that they are finally in active labor, they don't have the energy it takes to get through the long haul. It is great to sleep in between contractions, eat, stay hydrated (my favorite is coconut water or fresh watermelon) and take showers to help your body relax. As long as your water isn't broken, making love or intimate time with your partner is also quite a fabulous idea. This is not the time to invite the party in; oxytocin doesn't like a crowd. Women usually find themselves finishing up last minute details, shopping, or nesting about the house. When the real action starts, it is ideal to remove distractions, conversations, and settle in to the peaceful space you want to welcome your child into. Soft music, soft light, an environment that speaks to your individualized senses is the ideal space for you to delivery your baby.

FIRST STAGE OF LABOR, OR ACTIVE LABOR

Technically speaking, active labor is when a woman is dilated to 4cms and is having contractions that are rhythmically patterned around 4–5 minutes apart, are at least a minute long and have been that way for an hour. At this point, women are not usually speaking through contractions. And its best NOT to ask a laboring woman questions that require any cognitive thought, especially during the contraction itself. The function of labor requires that a woman be able to drop down into her limbic or primal mind, her animal mind. That part of her brain is only concerned with very short survival based thoughts like: thirst, cold, hot, pressure…. It is very difficult for a woman in active labor to express herself or to tend to the needs of those around her. If she is in any way engaged with her environment, you can assume it's still early. Moans and deep internal appearance, we are moving along! During this stage of labor, we encourage women to find their way through the sensations. Using a birth ball to rock on, especially draping your chest over it like on hand and knees, crawling, sitting on the toilet, and resting on the bed are great, or relaxing as much as possible. Some women find dancing or walking or even stomping around the house or outside in the garden to be extremely helpful. Also, a bath in active labor can utterly divine. If a woman likes to bathe prior to pregnancy, in labor the buoyancy can relive the sensations that accumulate just through the force of gravity. The key to this stage of labor is surrender: the more a woman can settle into or give herself over to the extraordinary sensations, tension just melts away and the body can do what it is designed to do.

As a typical rule, babies don't fall out unless this is a subsequent birth, however, I HAVE seen it happen for several first timers. If you feel like labor is going fast, pay more attention to the level of intensity rather than just the frequency. When labor pulls you so far in you are losing your connection to verbal (thinking) world around you, when all you can do is get down on the ground or lean against a hard surface and moan during a contraction, chances are likely that active labor has begun. There isn't a lot of talking going on, definitely not during a contraction, but even during the periods between contractions, women in active labor cannot hold a conversation. The deeper into active labor a woman goes, the more she is in a meditative state, occurring as if she is slipping into a semiconscious experience. Sometimes women will appear more like a wild animal. And, the truth is, there is no "right" way to do this. Every woman, like every baby, will find its way to come into this world and have its own birth story to tell.

SECOND STAGE OF LABOR OR PUSHING STAGE

Once a woman's cervix has completely dilated (10cms) and she feels the urge to push, it is time to get active in the birthing process. And it's also time to acknowledge how far we have come! In my opinion, women should prepare themselves for this next stage in the process by taking some deep breaths of renewed air, and let their baby know some big shifts are about to occur, that they are going to feel new sensations of pressure as he/she is being squeezed through the bones of the pelvis.

When there has been no pain medication administered, the sensation that rises up within a woman's body is unstoppable. I often say that it is like trying to stop a train. It is a force that spontaneously bursts from within and it is the body, coupled with a woman's own conscious efforts that move the child through the bones of the pelvis. For some women, pushing their child out is the most difficult part of the labor, quite possibly the hardest thing they have ever done in their lives. For others, it is a process of breathing the child down and looks more like an ecstatic experience. At this stage in labor, especially as the baby's head is beginning to emerge, a woman is filled to the absolute brim with hormones, deeply flooding her system. Unmedicated, this cascade of natural morphines and endorphins fill her, cross the placenta and also trigger the cellular memory of anyone in the room with her in such a way that everyone is getting contact high from the experience. To me, this flow or current of experience is crucial to keep intact. There is no reason to interfere with this beautiful process. Voices in the room should be kept to a whisper and any coaching of the process can be done with the deepest respect to the event at hand. This series of moments are ones that cant be redone and having a birth plan in advance for the wishes of the family should have been discussed with care providers and a common ground of understanding to have been reached PRIOR to the event. If the child should need some assistance in breathing or transitioning to the outside world, it should be done with the child still connected to its mother and oxygen supply through the umbilical cord. There are several studies that show the extraordinary effects of the blood perfusing to the baby through the cord. Babies will transition much quicker when they are held close and can feel the warmth and connection to their mother while hearing the welcoming voices they are familiar with. And most importantly, communication with the newborn as to what procedures are being done to them, why they are being done, and supporting them through the process by validating their experience through it will allow for them to be a participant in the process versus a victim of any procedure.

There is a tremendous amount of fear that can surface during this stage of labor. This is truly the doorway we must walk through alone as no one can do this part for us. All of our abuses, whether sexual or emotional tend to be stored here in our will center. It is such a worthy use of our energy to deal with any residual conversations, traumas, or blocks that might exist in our sacral and pelvic regions before the actual labor begins, or if possible, before the conception itself.

For those women whose mothers had a great experience of childbirth, the cellular memory and retelling of positive birth experiences lend themselves to an inherent openness and trust in the process, which generationally repeat in successive generations. The same is true for older siblings who witness the birth of younger ones. So often in interviews when meeting parents-to-be who were present at a homebirth as children, the absolute "normalness" of the birthing process is an experience they will never forget. This "normalness" has been lost, as our culture has stepped further into the state of technologically managing and manipulating the birth experience. The absolute sanctity, potential for personal empowerment, and opportunity for bonding is being adulterated by machines and bureaucratic systems that have no grasp on the loss, no connection to the impact on entire generations of individuals who now have come to fear birth and the prenatal period.

Stages of Labor, Dr. Robert Biter, MD

The process of labor is a dynamic one that is individual to every birth and every woman.

EARLY LABOR

The preparation of labor or early labor, may be seen as a time when the prostaglandins are changing and the cervix and uterus are ripening. This aspect of labor is the least understood and may very well be the reason that inductions frequently fail as providers attempt to recreate with medicine what we don't even understand in nature.

It is when the cervix starts to dilate and the contractions or surges are about 12–18 minutes apart and last around 20–30 seconds each. It's difficult to predict how long this could go on, as each pregnancy and birth is unique, but this could last for several hours.

ACTIVE LABOR

This is when the cervix is opening and shortening. During this time, the baby assists in her own way by following the cardinal movements of labor to make her way through the birth canal. The position of the baby during this time is also known as station where a provider estimates how close the baby is from a point in the mother's pelvic bone called the ischial spines.

During active labor, your cervix is most likely dilated to more than 4 centimeters and your contractions or surges are around every 3–5 minutes and last about 60 seconds.

TRANSITION LEADS TO THE PUSHING STAGE

This is typically when mothers assist their infant in moving through the cardinal movements to birth. The length of pushing is variable and can be affected by maternal positions, baby positioning, use of anesthesia and a variety of other factors. Of note, the *American College of Obstetrics and Gynecology Guidelines* for second stage, or the pushing stage, state that "length of second stage, in and of itself, is not an indication for shortening of the second stage" by forceps, vacuum, or Cesarean delivery.

During transition, you are likely 100 percent effaced and about 8–10 centimeters dilated. Your contractions or surges will be every 2 minutes and around 60–90 seconds in length. Pushing can take a few moments up to a few hours.

PLACENTA DELIVERY

Following the delivery of the baby, the placenta continues to provide nutrients until the umbilical cord stops pulsating and the placenta is then expelled. You will have actual contractions to "birth" the placenta and may consider keeping it to plant a tree in your baby's honor or have it dried out and turned into highly nutritional placenta pills which can help a great deal with recovery.

RECOVERY

The final stage involves recovery when the uterus returns to its non pregnant state and clamps down to prevent bleeding. Your midwife and possibly the nurses at a hospital will massage your uterus helping it to go back into its place shortly after birth. You may also pass a few fairly large blood clots and that is a normal part of the post birthing process.

ABOUT THE AUTHOR

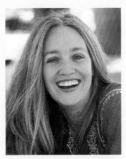

ANNI DAULTER, MSW, ecomama and author, has been a Conscious Family Living advocate and coach and an organic cook for many years, and has helped many families adopt a more natural and holistic approach to parenting and living. Anni developed Sacred Pregnancy classes to correspond with this book and a website for the pregnancy and mommy community. She has also partnered with Moby Wraps to create a postpartum Moby Wrap that helps women to naturally heal their bodies after birth.

Anni has been a guest speaker at Baby Celebration, The Pump Station, and several LA moms groups, has written for LA Parents and Orange County Parents, and is the resident baby/toddler-food expert for Hot Moms Club, City Mommy, Citibabes NY, Mindful Mama, Green Moms, and Macaroni Kid.

She lives in Philadelphia with her family—her son, Zoë (fourteen), her husband Tim, and their three children: daughter Lotus Sunshine (seven), little boy Bodhi (four), and baby boy River (one), all born happy and healthy either at home or in a birthing center.

www.annidaulter.com
www.sacredpregnancy.com

ABOUT THE PHOTOGRAPHERS

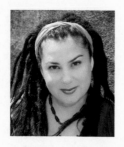

ELENA REGO is a prolific writer and photographer. Her work, which is deeply informed by her passion for women's spirituality and feminist theory, conveys the importance of engaging the spirit through making the mundane sacred and returning to the celebration of the rites of passages that mark our human lives.

Her writings have been included in various women's periodicals, including FoodPractice.com and the online magazine for this book, SacredPregnancy.com. Elena's artwork and photography have been shown in various galleries in Southern California, and she is currently writing her first book on the art of Food Practice.

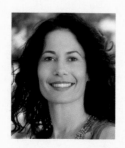

ALEXANDRA DEFURIO studied at UCLA and apprenticed with several fine art photographers before cultivating her own unique style. Her portraits are spontaneous and honest, invariably capturing their subjects' vulnerabilities and strengths. She creates images that are uncommonly authentic, revealing the essence as well as the form of the subject through what is for her an organic process. She lives in Santa Monica with her two favorite subjects—her daughters.